# ZERO BELLY
## COOKBOOK

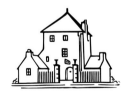

Ballantine Books
New York

# DAVID ZINCZENKO

# ZERO BELLY

## COOKBOOK

### 150+ Delicious Recipes
### to Flatten Your Belly,
### TURN OFF YOUR FAT GENES, and
### Help Keep You Lean for Life!

PHOTOGRAPHS BY JASON VARNEY

This book proposes a program of diet and exercise recommendations for the reader to follow. However, you should consult a qualified medical professional (and, if you are pregnant, your ob/gyn) before starting this or any other fitness program. Please seek your doctor's advice before making any decisions that affect your health or extreme changes in your diet, particularly if you suffer from any medical condition or have any symptom that may require treatment. As with any diet or exercise program, if at any time you experience any discomfort, stop immediately and consult your physician.

Published in the United States by Ballantine Books, an imprint of Random House, a division of Penguin Random House LLC, New York.

BALLANTINE and the HOUSE colophon are registered trademarks of Penguin Random House LLC.

LIBRARY OF CONGRESS CATALOGING-IN-PUBLICATION DATA
Zinczenko, David.
Zero belly cookbook : 150+ delicious recipes to flatten your belly, turn off your fat genes, and help keep you lean for life! /
David Zinczenko.
pages     cm
ISBN 978-1-101-96480-4 (hardback) — ISBN 978-1-101-96481-1 (ebook)
1. Reducing diets—Recipes. 2. Weight loss. 3. Abdomen—Muscles.
I. Title.
RM222.2.Z564 2015     641.5'635—dc23     2015022899

Printed in the United States of America on acid-free paper

randomhousebooks.com

987654321

First Edition

Book design by George Karabotsos
Photography by Jason Varney
Food styling by Carrie Purcell

To every chef who's ever picked up a spatula and thought, "How can I help myself and those I love to eat better today?" May this cookbook be among your most useful and beloved weapons in the battle for a healthier life.

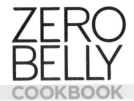

# Contents

# DISCOVER THE POWER OF ZERO BELLY

A Look at the Remarkable and Revolutionary **ZERO BELLY** Program, and the Stunning, Proven Health and Weight-Loss Benefits Behind It

Every once in a while, you read something that changes your life.

For some, it's a novel—*The Great Gatsby* perhaps, or *The Corrections*. For others, it's a motivational phrase, a memorable quote from Gandhi, or Lincoln, or Dr. King. But me, I'm a numbers guy.

And the numbers that rocked my world came from a study at Cambridge University a few years back. They're the numbers five and forty-seven.

As in, those of us who cook at home at least five times a week are 47 percent more likely to still be alive ten years from now.

As a guy who ate almost every meal at a restaurant, that study shook me to the core. As a man who lost his own father to obesity at a young age, and who struggled with his own weight for several years, it made sense. For most of our lives, you and I and almost everyone else in America have been giving control of our health, our weight, and our future to someone who doesn't even know who we are—and, frankly, doesn't care.

And we don't know who he is, either. But he probably works in a kitchen—in the back of a Chipotle, or a corner diner, or a McDonald's, or a nice Italian neighborhood restaurant. His job is to make our food as rich and tasty as he can, as cheaply as he can, with bargain-basement oils and unhealthy fats and plenty of added sugar, so we'll crave more, order more, and come back for more. How do all these fats and sugars and calories affect our health? That's not his problem.

But it's the problem you and I are going to solve together. *Zero Belly Cookbook* will show you how to seize control from the line cooks and food-lab technicians who rule your life, and put the power of food firmly in your grasp. The science is revolutionary. The results are irrefutable.

And the food? The food is just damn tasty.

# IT'S TIME TO TAKE CHARGE

*Zero Belly Cookbook* is going to change everything about how you eat, feel, and live. It will save you time, it will save you money, it will save you pounds—and in the end, it just might save your life.

I can say that, because I believe it's saved mine.

This book is the culmination of a lifetime spent hunting for an answer—an answer for one of the most vexing problems known to man. But it's much more than that. It's a celebration: a celebration of great food and the power it has to heal our bodies, soothe our souls, and give us back control of our lives. And it's a celebration of victory over the greatest health challenge of our times.

Steeped in decades of research, ZERO BELLY is unlike any

other weight-loss plan or recipe collection you've ever read. If you want to count calories, this book won't tell you how. If you want to deprive yourself of carbs or fats or any delicious region of the food map, go somewhere else. If you believe eating bland, boring food is the key to weight loss, then just close this book now and put it back on the shelf.

*The blueberry pancakes are great! Pancakes that are good for you and taste great? You can't beat that!*

—**MATT BRUNNER,** *44, lost 35 pounds and 6 inches from his waist*

But if you want to be on the front lines of a new revolution in weight loss, one that unlocks the power of food to rev up your metabolism, heal your digestive system, dramatically reduce your health risks, and literally turn "off" the genes that cause belly fat, then ZERO BELLY is the plan for you. The 150+ recipes in this book target belly fat directly, literally teaching your body how to lose weight quickly, and keep it off permanently, using the most delicious foods on the planet. It will do for you what it has done for thousands of fans who have joined the movement—*Zero Belly Diet* is a *New York Times* bestseller, international blockbuster, and social media phenomenon for a reason: It works for everyone.

And it will work for you.

# SOLVING THE RIDDLE—AT LAST

Belly fat—or "visceral fat," as the scientists call it—is the common link in almost every major health issue we face today. And for years, it had me in its grasp. Growing up an overweight kid, I watched as it slowly killed my father, its insidious and unrelenting grip unyielding to every effort he made to diet or exercise away the pounds. Its perfect storm of heart disease, diabetes, and high blood pressure finally took my father from me when he was just fifty-two. Looking in the mirror at my own round tummy, I knew one thing for certain: It was coming for me.

My life depended on finding an answer. Yours does, too. And ZERO BELLY gives us what we've been searching for all these years, finally: the answer.

It was the answer for June Caron, fifty-seven, who signed up to try the program and lost 12 pounds in just two weeks, shrinking from a size 12 to a size 5 in just one year. "My energy levels are increased, my routine medical tests for cholesterol, sugar levels, blood pressure all show great numbers, my stress levels are down, my confidence is up, my happiness is UP! I am finally off the diet roller coaster! Hail to the Chef!"

It was the answer for Jason Johnson, age forty, who lost 18 pounds and 3 inches off his waist in just five weeks. "I feel outstanding both mentally and physically. I recall exactly when this energy and mood shift hit me—it was on day three. I suddenly felt happy, almost euphoric, and my body told me I should just get up and start walking. I know it sounds corny, but it's true."

And it was the answer for Jean Connors, a retired elementary teacher who, at age seventy, happened to see me talking about my research on *Good Morning America*. Jean tried the plan and went

# SAFE AT HOME

**WHY LEARNING TO COOK IS THE SIMPLEST WAY TO SAVE YOUR OWN LIFE**

In March 2015, the U.S. Commerce Department reported that, for the first time in American history, spending in restaurants and bars had overtaken grocery store sales. That sea change has synced with our growing waistlines: As recently as 1992, we spent nearly twice as much in supermarkets as we did on dining out. And that trend is only likely to grow; people between the ages of twenty-five and thirty-four now spend nearly half as much on restaurant food as they do on rent! Here are six reasons to buck the trend and fire up the stove:

**You'll train yourself to eat smarter.** According to a Johns Hopkins study, people who cook at home not only consume fewer calories every single day, but they tend to consume fewer calories when they go to restaurants as well. The reason: cooking at home helps us understand portion control.

**You'll slash unwanted fat and sodium.** In an analysis of nineteen restaurant chains, researchers found that the average meal contained 151 percent of our recommended daily value for sodium, and almost half of all meals contained more than a full day's supply of fat.

**You'll feed your body the nutrients it needs.** According to research at Harvard University, families who ate at home together most days had higher intakes of calcium, fiber, iron, and vitamins $B_6$, $B_{12}$, C, and E; they also had lower overall saturated fat intakes.

**You'll raise a healthier family.** Children and adolescents who share family meals at home three or more times a week are more likely to be in a normal weight range and have healthier dietary and eating patterns than those who eat fewer home-cooked family meals.

**You'll eat the way your body wants you to.** Adults eat an average of 16 percent more food at restaurant meals, while kids eat an average of 52 percent more. The reason: larger serving plates and bowls trick our minds into thinking we should consume more.

**You'll keep your children safe.** Kids who eat fewer than three family meals a week are four times more likely to smoke, twice as likely to drink, and four times more likely to use drugs in the future, according to The National Center on Addiction and Substance Abuse at Columbia University.

from 142 pounds to a teenage-like 129—and dropped two pants sizes. "I really did not feel like I was on a diet," she says.

How can this plan work so quickly, so dramatically—and with such universal effectiveness? ZERO BELLY moves beyond calorie counting and deprivation, beyond self-denial and bland "diet" foods, and unlocks the power of real food—glorious, delicious, satisfying food—to turn off our fat genes and help us stay lean and healthy for life. The plan is based on nine key ZERO BELLY foods, which you'll read about on page 32, all of which work together to fight inflammation, reduce bloating, rev up your metabolism, and yes, actually turn off your fat genes and make weight loss automatic and effortless. And you'll learn how easy it is to prepare these ingredients with quick, simple, restaurant-quality recipes that will slim down your belly, not your wallet.

The emerging science around this approach was so new, and ZERO BELLY was so different from traditional "diets"—in fact, I hate even using that word!—that I knew I'd have to prove how its revolutionary approach worked. I assembled a test panel of eight hundred people who were eager to lose weight and convinced them to try this plan—one so radically different from traditional "diets" that at first many doubted it even was a "weight-loss" plan. Who loses weight eating burgers, sirloin steaks, chicken fajitas, and crab cakes—not to mention chocolate shakes?

My plan was to test the program for six weeks and measure the

*My wife says it's like living with a real chef now. Zero Belly makes eating healthy, simple, and delicious!*

**—BILL GRIESAU**, *34, lost 25 pounds*

results. But the testers didn't need six weeks. Within just fourteen days, some panelists had lost more than 16 pounds and more than 3 inches off their waist—without skipping meals, without giving up their favorite foods, without exercise, and without sacrificing one bit. And in the process, they dramatically—and measurably—improved their heart health and lowered their risk of diseases like diabetes.

This is what happens when you take control of your own food supply. There's no gimmick here, no silly trick: anything that sounds ridiculous, like adding butter to your coffee or living on peanut butter or banning foods invented after 10,000 BC, probably is ridiculous. All you really need is to learn a few simple recipes and center your meals around nine delicious foods—the fat-melting ZERO BELLY foods.

And that's what *Zero Belly Cookbook* will teach you to do.

# A BREAKTHROUGH IN THE BATTLE AGAINST BELLY FAT

I was gratified the test panelists lost weight, but I wasn't surprised. *Zero Belly Diet* and *Zero Belly Cookbook* are the result of a quarter century of meticulous research. As the creator of *Eat This, Not That!* and editorial director of *Men's Fitness* and *Shape* magazine, I've dedicated my career to studying the relationship between food and weight loss. I've personally investigated, tried, and—in most cases—debunked just about every dietary food trend that's come along in the last two decades, from low-fat eating to low-carb eating, from juicing to gluten-free to, yes, Paleo. (Show me a caveman who enjoyed steak frites with a nice glass of Merlot, and maybe I'll try that one again!)

For years, I've been hunting for the magic bullet in the battle against belly fat. Regular diet plans simply didn't work—either because they were too much effort (Who wants to turn everything they eat into juice?), or because they were too bland and hard to stick to (Watercress soup? I don't think so). Besides, when you "go on a diet," you eventually have to "go off" that diet, right? The whole weight-loss merry-go-round made no sense to me at all. My quest was to develop an eating plan that was as fun and delicious as it was healthy and effective.

A decade ago, I wrote *The Abs Diet,* which revolutionized the way we look at fat, and explained why targeting belly fat had to be everyone's number one health and weight-loss goal. But while that plan proved highly effective, it left a lot of questions unanswered: Why do some of us gain weight and others not, even when we eat the same amounts? And why, exactly, is carrying excess weight in your belly so dangerous?

And then there was the mystery of genetics, as personified by my best friend, my sworn enemy, my blood brother and childhood nemesis: my brother, Eric. Even as our father kept struggling with his weight, even as fat clung to my midsection like a baby kangaroo, Eric could seemingly eat anything he wanted without

*My favorite recipe was the chocolate cake. It felt so decadent and tasted amazing! Like cheating!*

**—JULISSA LOZA,** *44, lost 20 pounds and 4 inches from her waist*

gaining a pound of flab. I had "the fat genes," and there was nothing I could do about it. Meanwhile, Eric was a lean, fit, star athlete who won scholarships to college (and all the girls I'd had my eye on). "Fat genes?" Why me? Why not him? It didn't make sense! How can weight be "genetic" when it's also supposed to be about calories?

My research for *Zero Belly Diet* solved those mysteries and created a new weight-loss protocol that will work for everyone, including you—regardless of your health history, your lifestyle, or even your genes! (P.S. My brother is awesome.)

# THE POWER OF ZERO BELLY

Think back for a moment to the last meal that truly impressed you: a meal with flavors that seemed familiar yet somehow different from any other you had ever experienced. Not the familiar chain-restaurant fare, but something really unique: a home-cooked meal that looked so good on the plate, and felt so good in your mouth, that you wished that first bite could go on forever.

You may not have been thinking about it at the time, but beyond delighting your taste buds, chances are that meal did something else: It also helped inspire your body to shed belly fat. And while I knew from studying the science that the simple eating plan behind *Zero Belly Diet* would strip away belly fat rapidly and sustainably, what I didn't expect was just how rapid, and how dramatic, that weight loss would be—and how many additional benefits would come with following the ZERO BELLY protocol. Cooking the recipes in this book will give you status as the star chef in your neighborhood, and sometimes, that's enough. But they will also give you . . .

RIPPLING ABS! The amazing thing about ZERO BELLY is the rapid weight loss you'll experience—from your belly first. Panelists who took part in the first test run of ZERO BELLY reported up to 10 pounds gone in the first seven days, and some lost as much as 7 inches off their waist in just six weeks! ZERO BELLY flattens your stomach and reveals your abs quickly by reducing belly bloat and creating rapid fat metabolism; and it keeps weight off for the long term by quelling inflammation and turning off your fat-storage genes.

ETERNAL YOUTH! Okay, not exactly, but if you want to live a longer, healthier, richer life, the recipes in this book hold the key. In a mere six weeks on ZERO BELLY, you can slash your statistical risk of dying from diabetes, heart disease, or stroke by as much as 80 percent. That's because ZERO BELLY recipes are specifically designed to target the fat that matters most to your health: visceral fat—the kind that insinuates its way in and around your internal organs, pumping out inflammatory substances called adipokines, which raise your risk of all these diseases and more. According to the National Institutes of Health, women who carry excess fat around their waists are at greater risk of dying early from cancer or heart disease than women with smaller waistlines, even if they are of normal weight. For example, women with waist sizes equal to or greater than 35 inches are almost twice as likely to die of heart disease or cancer than women with a waist size of less than 28 inches, regardless of their actual weight or body mass index.

UNSTOPPABLE GENIUS! According to researchers at Rush University Medical Center, the protein responsible for metabolizing fat in the belly is the same protein found in the hippocampus, the part of the brain that controls memory and learning. People with higher levels of abdominal fat actually have depleted this fat-metabolizing protein, making them 3.6 times more likely to suffer from memory loss and dementia later in life.

But a few years ago, scientists discovered something even more ominous: They performed CT scans on a large number of healthy, middle-aged men and women to measure their visceral fat. They also used the same technology to determine their total brain

# THE SULTAN OF SPICE

**MEET THE MAN WHO BUILT THE LIFE-ALTERING RECIPES IN THIS BOOK**

In a cavernous kitchen in New York's Tribeca neighborhood, a lean gent in white sits at a table set for twenty, scribbling feverishly on cocktail napkins.

"Oats." He taps his pen on the table with one hand and thumbs his wedding band with the other. "What about a play on grits? Yeah, yeah." He grabs a notepad from his pocket, flips to a clean page, and writes down a short list of ingredients. This is thirty-five-year-old Jason Lawless, executive chef at White Street restaurant in New York, and he's playing a game of poker with the **ZERO BELLY** ingredients, mixing and matching them to find the best possible hand to play.

"Would I eat this if I wasn't on a diet?" he asks himself of his new idea, as if to vet his own creative impulse. "Absolutely. Would my wife eat this? Yes. And would my sons eat this?" He crosses out two ingredients. "That's gonna be killer."

Like me, Jason grew up the child of a single mother. But whereas I gravitated to fast food—and became a nutrition expert to overcome my girth—Jason went the other way. He became a chef.

"It actually started when I was five or six," Jason says of his passion for cooking. "My mom worked a lot, so at a young age if I was hungry I had to cook for myself." Fast-forward some fifteen years and Jason's natural ability would see him graduate from the Scottsdale Culinary Institute of Arizona with a degree that led him to Star Canyon in Dallas, where he was hired as chef de partie, and then to Manhattan, where he found work at the Indian-inspired restaurant Tabla, learning a whole new world of spices and flavors. Jason went on to work at successful NYC restaurants including Alain Ducasse's Mix and Café Gray—an experience he says proved the most influential of his career. "We used food from all over the world." He also served as executive chef at the AAA Three Diamond Woodstock Inn and Resort in Vermont. Then, in 2014, he joined top chef Floyd Cardoz to build the critically acclaimed menu at White Street, where he currently serves as executive chef.

"We don't use butter or cream at White Street," says Jason. "Eating healthy doesn't have to be boring or complicated. My hope is that anyone who picks up this book finds a **ZERO BELLY**–approved version of all their favorite dishes, plus a few new ones that become healthy family traditions."

THREE ADJECTIVES THAT JASON USES TO DESCRIBE HIS FOOD PHILOSOPHY:
*"Seasonal, elegant, simple."*

FAVORITE *ZERO BELLY COOKBOOK* RECIPE:
*"Black Pepper Shrimp with Creamy Oats, Cherry Tomatoes, and Asparagus" (page 128).*

TOP TIP FOR MAKING HEALTHY FOOD TASTE GOOD:
*"Fresh herbs add flavor and complexity to any dish and are a great substitute for salt and calorie-dense sauces."*

FAVORITE *ZERO BELLY COOKBOOK* INGREDIENT:
*"I keep a jar of Black Pepper Marinade (page 239) in the fridge. It's good on everything and full of healing spices with proven health benefits."*

volume. And what they learned was that the more visceral fat a person had, the less brain mass they had. If that's not enough to spark you into action, consider this: In a study at Georgia Regents University, researchers took mice that had been genetically bred to be obese and diabetic, put them on exercise programs to lose weight, and surgically removed their remaining belly fat. The mice were then tested for memory and brain function, and actually found to be smarter than they had been before the weight loss. This may be the closest we ever get to owning Warren Buffet's secret playbook!

# VAST WEALTH! In a study in the *International Journal of Obesity*, researchers gave participants a series of résumés with small photos of the applicants attached. What they learned was that starting salary, leadership potential, and hiring decisions were impacted negatively when the photo showed a person who was overweight—most severely in the case of obese women. Another study, by researchers at the University of Florida, found that based on these prejudices, an overweight woman who works for twenty-five years will wind up with an average of $389,300 less than a thinner one.

# EVERLASTING HAPPINESS!
ZERO BELLY recipes are packed with mood-enhancing nutrients like folate, a vitamin found in leafy greens and legumes. But more important, by balancing your gut health, they bring order to the area of the body where more than 90 percent of our "feel good" hormone, serotonin, is stored. As a result, you'll feel less stress and anxiety: In studies, women with visceral fat accumulation have been shown to have elevated secretions of cortisol, a stress hormone, and an increased sensitivity to stress hormones along the hypothalamus, pituitary, and adrenal glands.

And new research from the British journal *Age and Ageing* indicates that losing belly fat may be the most significant thing you can do to improve your life as you get older. In a study, researchers surveyed nearly six hundred men between the ages of sixty and seventy-four, asking them about a wide range of issues, from their physical health to their social lives to their mental and emotional well-being. Then the researchers measured their testosterone levels and, using X-rays and MRIs, measured their visceral and subcutaneous fat levels as well. What they discovered was that the greatest single factor impacting quality of life was visceral fat—the less belly fat these men had, the more likely they were to report being happy with their lives.

And now, you can get all of this and more—just by cooking these delicious recipes! ZERO BELLY: You'll come for the abs. You'll stay for the health, wealth, and happiness.

# WHAT TO EXPECT WHEN YOU EAT THE ZERO BELLY WAY

Beating belly fat is the goal. **ZERO BELLY** is the path to victory. But no road was ever carved out by a single person. When I first developed this program, I put together a test panel of more than eight hundred people, men and women who provided living, breathing proof of the effectiveness of this breakthrough plan. More important, they also provided critical feedback that helped me make it better. Their success can be your success.

What we learned from the test panel is that **ZERO BELLY** works much more quickly than a typical weight-loss regimen. By attacking digestive issues and inflammation at the same time that it melts fat and builds muscle, my plan creates a four-prong attack on visceral fat that's unlike anything else out there. And by targeting your fat genes with a protocol designed to switch them to "off," it helps you maintain and continue your weight-loss journey for a lifetime.

Here's a week-by-week breakdown of what happened to our test panel—and what you can expect from week one on **ZERO BELLY**.

# WEEK ONE: LOOK AND FEEL LIGHTER—IMMEDIATELY

The first thing you'll notice on this program—within a few days, in most cases—is that your pants will fit better, you'll look leaner, and you'll feel less bloated and lighter. You'll step on the scale and wonder if this is a trick; while you may lose up to six pounds in the first week, you'll feel like you've lost a lot more.

That's because the first thing ZERO BELLY affects is your digestion, helping to balance your gut health, reduce bloating, and fight inflammation. It's step one in your attack on belly fat: You're prepping your body for dramatic weight loss. Your belly will almost immediately look leaner, and you'll notice a huge spike in energy and emotional well-being.

Martha Chesler, fifty-four, is an Ohio-based teacher and mother of three adult children. She had tried any number of weight-loss plans, from meal replacement plans to formal work-out plans like Curves. But she was dissatisfied with her tummy, and when she heard about ZERO BELLY, it sounded like a great opportunity.

"I saw results immediately," she says. "I felt better physically and emotionally and wanted to keep that feeling going." Bryan Wilson, twenty-nine, a bachelor in beautiful Monument, Colorado, had the same experience. "Almost immediately I lost the bloat," he says. And Bob McMicken, fifty-one, from Lancaster, California, reports looking and feeling flatter "within days." The same goes for Fred Sparks, from Katy, Texas: "I noticed results in the first week," says the thirty-nine-year-old emergency-response adviser and father of two. "I felt much less bloating and digesting problems. It really was amazing."

That kind of immediate result is great if you've got a pool party or a college reunion coming up in a week. But we're hunting bigger game here—an all-out war on belly fat. Fortunately, the results keep getting better!

# WEEK TWO: SUDDEN, EFFORTLESS WEIGHT LOSS

When June Caron got on the scale at the beginning of week two, she was stunned: six pounds gone in the first seven days. "And the weight just keeps coming off," she says. The fifty-five-year-old work-control specialist from North Oxford, Massachusetts, had begun to gain weight in her belly—the very thing that puts postmenopausal women at the same elevated risk for heart disease as men. It was a health crisis that needed attacking, but June had seen a lot of other weight-loss strategies fail—Weight Watchers, workout DVDs, you name it. "I've joined gyms, but rarely stuck with them," she confesses. Now, she finally had a plan that would not only help her manage her weight, but her health as well.

Matt Brunner, a forty-three-year-old professor in Glenside, Pennsylvania, who had seen only mediocre results from past weight-loss plans, experienced the same thing: seven pounds gone in just a week.

At the same time, back in Ohio, Martha Chesler was down 10 pounds within the first ten days, and starting to notice something else as well—her own health was improving measurably. During a checkup with her chiropractor, she discovered her heart was suddenly functioning much more efficiently. During a fitness test using a stationary cycle, where her heart rate would normally climb to 112 beats per minute within minutes of starting on the bike, she found an enormous change: "During the workout I could not raise my heart rate over 96 bmp! It was great to know good things were happening that I couldn't even see."

## WEEK THREE: OLD CLOTHES BECOME NEW AGAIN

Krista Kirk, thirty-three, was always self-conscious about her belly, and when people started asking her if she was pregnant (she wasn't), she knew something had to change. Atkins, Nutrisystem— you name the plan, Krista can give the review: boring and ineffective. But after two weeks on the program, Krista's pants began to feel looser, her hips slimmed down—and she was finally able to dress in a way that reflected her true sense of style: "I'd avoided wearing high heels because the extra weight made my knees hurt so bad. I can actually wear my heels with confidence and without pain!"

In Pennsylvania, Matt Brunner was having the same experience. "My clothes got too big. My 'skinny' clothes all looked good again."

## WEEK FOUR: SCULPT YOUR NEW BODY

After a high-risk pregnancy during which she was unable to do more than walk, thirty-eight-year-old Jennie Joshi had been working hard to lose her baby weight. But the corporate sales trainer and mother of two simply couldn't get rid of her "pregnancy pooch." Low-carb, high-protein—you name the diet, Jennie had tried it. But the belly-specific, targeted approach of ZERO BELLY was different. She dropped 11 pounds in just about four weeks, but more important, she lost them where she wanted to lose them: "The pregnancy pooch is leaving!" she says. "I feel like the old pre-baby Jennie is back!"

Sticking to a weight-loss plan isn't easy for a working mom with two small children, and that's what impressed her about my program the most: The healthy recipes gave Jennie plenty of family-friendly options that even her foodie husband enjoyed. "ZERO BELLY is easy to follow regardless of life's demands. It's not a cleanse or a fad diet, it's a lifestyle."

And the fast results help keep you motivated. "I met a group of co-workers who hadn't seen me in a month, and they were all astonished at the differences they could see in me," says Jennie. "They wanted to know what I was doing."

It's at week four that the body-sculpting aspects of the protocol really begin to take effect. Beyond the flatter belly, most subjects also reported a leaner overall look. "My arms lost some of their flab, and my shoulders, biceps, and triceps tightened up," says Bryan. And the other side effects of the plan aren't bad either.

"My energy is at a very high level, whereas before ZERO BELLY I was feeling tired all the time," says June Caron. "My skin and nails look better. I'm sleeping better. Everyone says I look much younger!"

# WEEK FIVE:
## SAVE YOUR OWN LIFE

Katrina Bridges, of Bethalto, Illinois, wanted to lose weight and shrink her belly. But what she didn't know when she started ZERO BELLY was that she entered the test panel with a dramatically elevated risk of heart disease and diabetes. Based on Katrina's starting weight of 237, and her waist circumference of 50 inches, we were able to calculate that her risk of dying from heart attack, stroke, or complications of diabetes was 90 percent greater than that of the general population.

In five weeks, that all changed. Katrina stripped off 12 pounds quickly, but more important, she shed five inches off her waistline. Thanks to a risk calculator known as A Body Shape Index (ABSI), we can measure her exact progress; in just five weeks, Katrina reduced her elevated risk from these diseases by a whopping 80 percent. And, she says, "I just felt like I had more overall strength throughout my body."

Meanwhile, Martha Chesler was not only experiencing a healthier heart, but something else: an end to her heartburn. "My acid reflux is under control, with minimum medication," she reported. And studies show heartburn isn't just an annoyance; like elevated belly fat, heartburn is a risk factor for certain types of cancer.

## WEEK SIX: DRAMATIC CHANGES THAT LAST

I don't like to think of ZERO BELLY as a "weight-loss" plan, although you'll lose a lot of weight. I like to think of it as a plan to shrink your waist and improve your life. So I get excited by stories like that of Kyle Cambridge of Peace River, Alberta, Canada, who lost four inches off his waist—and 25 pounds of fat—in just six weeks. "I even had to buy a new belt!" he said. "But the best was when Stacie [my wife] came up to me in the kitchen, and gave me a hug. She laughed and smiled and said, 'I can wrap my hands around you again.'"

June Caron lost 4 inches off her waist in just six weeks. Fred Sparks stripped off 5 inches and 21 pounds of fat. Bob McMicken (down 24 pounds) and Bryan Wilson (19 pounds gone) both shed six inches. And Martha Chesler lost 21 pounds and seven inches off her waist in less than forty days. And they all remarked on how easy and effective the program was.

"The food was so tasty," says Krista. "I love the ZERO BELLY Drinks," says Bob.

"It has been beyond comparison to any other diet or exercise program I have ever tried. I am never, ever hungry," says June.

These people discovered the amazing benefits of ZERO BELLY, and they did it without feeling hungry, tired, or overwhelmed.

In the coming pages, I'll show you how you can, too!

# ZERO BELLY

My plan targets the fat that matters most—visceral belly fat—through a unique nutritional approach powered by the latest revolutionary research in weight loss, digestive health, and anti-inflammatory foods. Here are the basics:

## MEALS

Three square meals; one **ZERO BELLY** Drink; and one snack per day.

## NUTRIENTS

While **ZERO BELLY** is carefully balanced to give you all the essential nutrients you need to strip away fat and reveal lean, healthy muscle, you'll ask three important **ZERO BELLY** questions before each meal or snack:

- **Where's my protein?**
- **Where's my fiber?**
- **Where's my healthy fat?**

## FOODS

**Z**ERO BELLY Drinks (high-protein and delicious)

**E**ggs

**R**ed Fruits

**O**live Oil and Other Healthy Fats

**B**eans, Rice, Oats, and Other Healthy Fiber

**E**xtra Plant Protein

**L**ean Meats and Fish

**L**eafy Greens, Green Tea, and Bright Vegetables

**Y**our Favorite Spices

# STARTER KIT

## LIMIT

Processed foods; saturated fat; sugar; refined grains; wheat; dairy.

## MAXIMIZE

High-phytonutrient, high-fiber fruits, vegetables, legumes, and grains; lean sources of protein; mono- and polyunsaturated fats; omega-3 fatty acids.

## DRINKS

One snack a day will be a **ZERO BELLY** Drink, a satisfying plant-based, protein-filled smoothie.

## SPECIAL DIETARY CONCERNS

**ZERO BELLY** is not strictly gluten-free, dairy-free, or vegan, but I've built this program specifically with those dietary concerns in mind. **ZERO BELLY** reduces your exposure to gluten and dairy while boosting plant-based sources of protein. Those searching for gluten-free, dairy-free, or vegan diet plans can easily adapt **ZERO BELLY** to fit their needs.

## ALCOHOL

Limit alcohol to no more than one drink per day during the initial six weeks of the program.

## EXERCISE

To turbocharge the effects of **ZERO BELLY**, I invite you to try the **ZERO BELLY** Workouts, a unique full-body fitness experience that builds ab muscles while simultaneously toning your entire body. There is no other workout plan like it! You'll find the complete training program in *Zero Belly Diet* and in the **ZERO BELLY** app.

# CHAPTER ONE

# ZERO BELLY TURBO-CHARGED

The Four-Point Plan for Turning Off Your Fat
Genes and Keeping You Lean for Life

Sometimes you start out to write a book, and you accidentally start a revolution.

Within just weeks after the publication of *Zero Belly Diet*, a spontaneous support group, Zero Belly Way of Life, sprung up on Facebook, with readers swapping recipes, sharing tips, and describing their experiences as they watched stubborn pounds suddenly fall away, effortlessly. In fact, readers have become my best advertisers, sharing word of mouth about how effective ZERO BELLY is. They've just had one consistent request:

Can we have more recipes, please?

This cookbook is a delicious answer to those tens of thousands of clamoring fans who want to take ZERO BELLY to the next level. ZERO BELLY—like the Facebook group says—isn't a diet. It's a way of life. And the more seamlessly you can incorporate its principles into your day-to-day routine, the greater the health gains and weight loss you'll experience.

If you're not already a fan of ZERO BELLY, this chapter will give you some background into the program: how it works and, more interesting, why it works. Even if you don't care much for science (hey, I'm here to get some awesome recipes!), you'll find this little recap pretty cool, because it explains why simply tweaking the way in which we eat can change everything about our bodies and our lives. (And I bet the Slow-Cooked Beef Stew on page 149 is going to taste that much more delicious when you know just how many great things it's doing for your body.)

# FOUR WAYS THESE RECIPES TURBOCHARGE WEIGHT LOSS

Ask anyone what the key principles of weight loss are, and they'll probably come back with something like "hunger, sweat, and misery." Between the toothy TV trainers who want to take you to boot camp and the supplement companies who want to sell you "fat-burners" and the diet food makers who've packaged up low-fat, low-carb, low-cal, low-fun frozen misery meals, it's no wonder that dropping pounds seems like it has to be ugly and onerous.

But that's because most weight-loss plans are based on the erroneous idea that cutting calories is the way to strip off pounds. Or that cutting fat, or carbs, or meat, is the golden path. Or that pounding away at the treadmill or the stationary rower is the way to go. And all of those approaches will work, to a certain extent. But each of them comes with the same three problems:

- **They're really hard.**
- **They're not sustainable in the long run.**
- **They work against your body, not with it.**

ZERO BELLY is something different. ZERO BELLY tweaks your approach to eating in a way that makes weight loss effortless. It resets your metabolism so fat-burning becomes automatic. And it harnesses the power of food to work with your body, unleashing your natural weight-loss mechanisms. I don't have to convince you that losing belly fat is a good idea.

We just have to convince your body.

If you carry more fat than you want, it's because your body has programmed itself to store the energy you eat as fat. Your body is like one of those crazy hoarders whose every nook and cranny is crammed with stuffed cats and dusty flea market finds. All that exercise and diet can do are to tidy up a bit. But if we can convince your body to give up all the energy it's storing as fat, you'll see rapid changes that will last a lifetime. It's like backing the 1-800-GOT-JUNK truck up to your door and unloading all the unwanted storage!

In fact, when I built the original *Zero Belly Diet,* I identified three ways in which the program works. But since its publication in December 2014, we've learned even more about the power of the ZERO BELLY Foods, and new ways to tweak the program to turbocharge your weight loss.

## ZERO BELLY PRINCIPLE #1:
# BOOST METABOLISM

The first thing ZERO BELLY does is to turn up the dial on your internal calorie furnace—a furnace that feeds on belly fat. ZERO BELLY unleashes the power of protein, fiber, and healthy fats to burn calories by encouraging lean muscle growth and maximizing the thermogenic effects of eating—meaning, the number of calories you burn simply by digesting your food.

You've probably heard a lot about "fat-burning foods," but how exactly do they work? In fact, there are two types of fat-burning foods: those that decrease blood sugar spikes (when your blood sugar spikes, the hormone insulin rushes in and tries to store the sugar calories as fat), and those that increase metabolism (meaning you literally burn off more calories, even as you sleep).

The key is to attack fat from both ends—prevent more from forming while burning off the stores you already have. Foods that control blood sugar generally contain some combination of protein, healthy fat, and fiber—the three hallmarks of a ZERO BELLY meal. Calorie-burning foods, on the other hand, include green tea, vinegar, and anything that's high in protein such as eggs, lean meats, and fish.

Protein also helps build lean muscle tissue—belly fat's sworn enemy. In fact, the more muscle your body has, the more belly fat it burns on a daily basis. And the more belly fat you have, the harder it is to maintain muscle mass. That's why lean protein and other muscle-supporting foods are such a critical component of these recipes.

## ZERO BELLY TURBOCHARGE >
## Add a cup of green tea each day.

Protein, fiber, and healthy fats are all found throughout these recipes, but adding a cup (or two) of green tea to your daily regimen can help fire your fat furnace in both ways. First, it controls blood sugar and quashes hunger: In a Swedish study that looked at green tea's effect on hunger, researchers divided up participants into two groups. One group sipped water with their meal and the other group drank green tea. Not only did tea-sippers report less of a desire to eat their favorite foods (even two hours after sipping the brew), they found those foods to be less satisfying. And second, it boosts your calorie burn, especially if you have it before any type of exercise: In a recent twelve-week study, participants who combined a daily habit of 4 to 5 cups of green tea each day with a 25-minute sweat session lost an average of two more pounds than the non-tea-drinking exercisers. Once again it's the power of the unique catechins found in green tea that can blast adipose tissue by triggering the release of fat from fat cells (particularly in the belly), and then speeding up the liver's capacity for turning that fat into energy. All this while doing something unique for your heart: A 2015 study from the Institute of Food Research found that the polyphenols in green tea block a "signaling molecule" called VEGF, which in the body can trigger both heart disease and cancer.

## ZERO BELLY PRINCIPLE #2:
# HEAL YOUR GUT

Happening right now, inside your belly, is an epic power struggle worthy of Shakespeare. But instead of Tudors and Plantagenets, you have different sorts of microbes battling it out to become monarch of your midsection—about five hundred different tribes, in fact. Some of them break down your food and extract nutrients; others hunt for food pathogens that snuck in on a bad bit of bratwurst; still others help protect you from colds and flus. (In fact, 80 percent of our immune system is based in our guts.) Scientists even believe that depression may be caused in part by unbalanced gut microbes, since 95 percent of our feel-good hormone serotonin is also located in the belly.

But it's our weight that's most dramatically affected by these little buggers. In fact, studies show that obese people have higher levels of bad bacteria from the phylum Firmicutes, while lean people have higher levels of bacteria from the phylum Bacteroidetes. How critical is a healthy gut to weight loss? Researchers at Kyung Hee University in Seoul, Korea, induced obesity in lab rats by feeding them a high-fat diet, then fed one group of them probiotics (in this case, *Lactobacillus brevis,* a healthy bacteria found in fermented foods like kimchi). The probiotic suppressed the diet-induced increase in weight gain by 28 percent!

But as with any conflict, sometimes the good guys get overwhelmed. Too much junk food (especially sugar) can knock our digestive systems out of whack and give the advantage over to the Firmicutes (a poorly named tribe, as they make you neither firm nor cute); so too can drugs such as antibiotics, heartburn remedies, or antidepressants. That's why ZERO BELLY Foods are high in fiber and low in sugar, preservatives, and bloating foods like dairy. When you're feeling lean and clean, it means your belly is in balance and the good guys are ruling the day.

## ZERO BELLY TURBOCHARGE >
## Give your belly biome a workout.

One of the big buzzwords in nutrition right now is "resistant starch." No, it's not something your dry cleaner sprays on your shirt to make it wrinkle less. It's actually a type of carbohydrate that, as the name suggests, resists digestion.

A lot of the buzz around resistant starch is about its great metabolism-boosting properties—in fact, it hits both ends of the metabolism spectrum, slowing down your digestive process (thereby controlling blood sugar) while also forcing your body to burn more calories during the digestion process. But resistant starch has another awesome ZERO BELLY property: it feeds your "good" belly bacteria.

When you do resistance training, your muscles get stronger. But according to a 2015 study in the *Journal of Functional Foods,* when you eat resistant starch, your gut biome gets stronger—healthy bacteria literally get a workout digesting the healthy starch, becoming more dominant and leading to a healthier gut.

# ZERO BELLY PRINCIPLE #3:
# COOL INFLAMMATION

You know what happens when the gums around your teeth get red and irritated, right? That's inflammation, caused by the wrong kind of bacteria building up around your mouth. Well, when your belly bacteria get out of whack, they start to irritate the lining of your digestive system in much the same way. And in recent years, we've learned just how huge a roll this process plays in weight gain.

Once the bad bugs start taking control in your gut, the inflammation that begins in your digestive tract spreads to other parts of your body. Think of the lining of your belly like a fine screen. When bacteria get out of whack, they begin to irritate the lining of the intestines, and the holes in the screen become larger. Bacteria, food particles, and other nasty things escape your GI tract and get into your bloodstream, where they begin to attack the body. The body fights back with inflammation, leading to weight gain and bloating, and putting you at greater risk for everything from asthma and allergies to diabetes and heart disease.

Since the publication of *Zero Belly Diet*, new research has shown us not only that inflammation throughout the body is unhealthy, but that our belly fat itself can become inflamed, raising our risk of a host of diseases, but most specifically diabetes. In fact, early in 2015, Australian and Japanese researchers found they could reverse diabetes by dampening the inflammatory response in fat tissues. In a study in the journal *Nature Immunology*, the researchers revealed that in healthy people, fat has its own specialized immune cells, called regulatory T cells, or "Tregs." These Tregs act like guardians of our immune system, protecting us from the inflammation that's related to diabetes and arthritis. But when obesity sets in, the Tregs actually disappear from our fat cells. "The fat tissue of obese people has lower numbers of Tregs than the fat tissue of people in a healthy weight range," the researchers explained. "We can no longer think of fat tissue simply as energy storage. Fat tissue is increasingly being recognized as a crucial organ that releases hormones" and plays a key role in decreasing disease.

## ZERO BELLY TURBOCHARGE >
# Double down on plant protein.

In a 2015 study in the *Journal of Diabetes Investigation*, researchers discovered that patients who ingested higher amounts of vegetable protein were far less susceptible to metabolic syndrome (a disease that ought to be renamed "diabolic syndrome"—it's basically a combination of high cholesterol, high blood sugar, and obesity). That means that eating whole foods from vegetables—and supplementing with vegan protein powder—is one of the best ways to keep extra weight at bay. A second study in *Nutrition Journal* found that "plant protein intakes may play a role in preventing obesity."

ZERO BELLY Drinks are made specifically with plant protein, but to add more into your day, focus on vegetable protein sources such as lentils, hemp or chia seeds, quinoa, nuts, seeds, and beans. Or try adding spirulina to your smoothies; it's one of the few plant foods that are mostly protein by weight (about 70 percent).

## ZERO BELLY PRINCIPLE #4:
# TURN OFF YOUR FAT GENES

In a 2014 study in the *International Journal of Obesity*, researchers studied a group of men and women who all shared a similar BMI. Through a series of medical tests, they broke the group into two sets: one metabolically healthy, and a second that showed elevated total cholesterol, higher LDL (bad) cholesterol, and reduced insulin sensitivity (a precursor to diabetes). Since they all had similar body weights, what was the difference between the two groups? Those in the unhealthy group had more actively expressed genes for inflammation.

And in a giant study in the journal *Nature,* scientists scoured the DNA libraries of more than three hundred thousand people, constructing the largest-ever genetic map of obesity, and determined that at least 20 percent of our excess body weight is caused by the action of our genes.

In a 2015 study in *Obesity Reviews*, researchers explained that our body weight is determined in part by a "set point" that's programmed by energy balance circuitry in the hypothalamus and other specific brain regions. That set point is determined by our genes, but exposure to an "obesogenic environment"—being surrounded by junk food—can cause that set point to drift upward.

## ZERO BELLY TURBOCHARGE >
## Add some red wine to your diet.

Have a glass of red wine or two a week. It could help you burn fat better, according to a 2015 study in *Nutritional Biochemistry*. Over a 10-week trial, mice that got the human equivalent of about one and a half cups of red grapes a day accumulated less abdominal fat, and had lower blood sugar, than those that didn't—even though both sets of furry subjects were being fed high-fat diets. In fact, the ellagic acid in the grapes lowered the fat mice's blood sugar to nearly the same levels as lean, normally fed mice.

Red wine is the best possible source of a micronutrient called resveratrol, which works on the genes responsible for obesity and liver steatosis—essentially, belly fat that forms around your liver. That's because resveratrol is found primarily in the skin of grapes, and the alcohol in wine draws the resveratrol out of the skins, creating a concentrated dose that's greater than just grape juice. (You know how, if you leave a splash of wine sitting in a glass overnight, you get a flaky burgundy deposit at the bottom? That's resveratrol.)

# CHAPTER TWO

# THE ZERO BELLY FOODS

Nine Startling Superfoods That Will Change Your Body and Your Life—in Just Fourteen Days!

Sensuous.

Enticing.

Decadent.

Delicious.

These are not the words one typically associates with a "diet" cookbook. But ZERO BELLY is no ordinary diet, and this is no ordinary cookbook.

It is, instead, a journey through some of the world's most startling flavors and most satiating foods—some of them comforting, some of them refreshing, and all of them utterly irresistible.

How can a cookbook based on a bestselling diet possibly sit on the same shelves as the highest-level gourmet offerings? And how can food this rich, this scrumptious, possibly help you lose weight, regain your health, and improve every aspect of your life?

First, the science of ZERO BELLY is the science of flavor. This is an eating plan that focuses on taste, because the taste of a food is the single strongest indicator that it has the power to unlock your metabolism, heal your body, even turn off the genes responsible for weight gain. Sweet, moist fruits; deep, decadent chocolate; bright, crunchy vegetables; soulful, smoky meats; and rich, silky oils are the backbone of the ZERO BELLY eating plan, each enhanced with herbs and spices that are as potent on your plate as they are inside your body. The ZERO BELLY plan harnesses the power of real food to target belly fat—the most dangerous type of fat there is—by unlocking your body's own natural fat burners.

And second, because the man who helped create most of these 150+ recipes is one of the most inventive, exciting young chefs in America today: Jason Lawless, executive chef at White Street in New York's Tribeca neighborhood, and a culinary artist who specializes in making simple flavors dance on your tongue like a Bollywood cast of thousands.

Plus, I've included special recipes from some of the most celebrated chefs in America—folks like Anita Lo of Annisa in New York; Seamus Mullen of El Colmado Butchery; and California cuisine pioneer Susan Feniger—and even a handful from the ZERO BELLY fans who've taken the principles of this plan and added their own unique and flavorful twists.

If you are here to experience dramatic, sustainable weight loss, you have come to the right place. And if you are here to enjoy some of the most exciting and inventive recipes ever assembled—recipes that are as quick and easy as they are enticing—then guess what? You've still come to the right place.

When I challenged Chef Jason to create these special ZERO BELLY recipes, I gave him a few parameters that I thought might make him flinch. First, the recipes needed to conform to a light set of rules: while ZERO BELLY isn't gluten-free or dairy-free, neither of these foods should be part of most recipes. I wanted a plan that would work for anyone, even those who struggle with gluten allergies or lactose intolerance (both of which can lead to bloating and, as a result, weight gain). Second, he needed to base his recipes around the most potent foods on the planet—foods that were proven to attack belly fat and turn off the genes responsible for weight gain.

He didn't flinch.

While we've included a few Zero Guilt Cheat Meals that include small amounts of dairy (a fan of cheese, I couldn't resist requesting a decadent lasagna!), they're clearly marked, should you choose to adhere strictly to the **ZERO BELLY** guidelines.

The **ZERO BELLY** Foods are so naturally delicious, and lend themselves so easily to great cooking, that making brilliant recipes was a snap for a master like Jason. Here are the foods I challenged him to embrace—the foods that are about to change your life.

# ZERO BELLY DRINKS
## Maximize Nutritional Intake

To experience the full impact of the **ZERO BELLY** program, each day you should supplement your regular meals with one of the blended smoothie drinks you'll find starting on page 214. These drinks are so delicious, and so easy to make, that you can have them for breakfast, as a snack, as a meal replacement, or even as a dessert. Studies show that high-protein, low-fat smoothies are highly effective at rushing nutrients into your body, particularly your muscles.

I've stripped all the **ZERO BELLY** Drink recipes of the dairy, added sugars, and artificial ingredients so common in popular commercial shakes, and packed them with real fruits, nuts, vegan proteins, and dairy alternatives like almond and coconut milks. Why the alternative milks? First, dairy can be difficult to digest for some folks—and poor digestion leads to inflammation, which leads to weight gain. But there's more to it than that: In 2014, Swedish scientists at Uppsala University found that women who drank three or more glasses of milk a day died at nearly twice the rate of those who drank less than one glass a day. Broken bones were more common in women who were heavy milk drinkers as well. While this is only a preliminary study, it's further reason why using non-dairy milk in your daily smoothie is a wise move.

# Eggs
## Turn Off Visceral Fat Genes

Eggs are the single best dietary source of the B vitamin choline, an essential nutrient used in the construction of all the body's cell membranes. Choline deficiency is linked directly to the genes that cause visceral fat accumulation, particularly in the liver. Yet according to a 2015 National Health and Nutrition Examination Survey, only a small percentage of all Americans eat daily diets that meet the U.S. Institute of Medicine's Adequate Intake of 425 mg for women and 550 mg for men.

# Red Fruits
## Turn Off Obesity Genes

Like professional basketball players, all fruits are good at what they do. But a red hue is a sign that your snack is just that little bit better—watermelon is to honeydew what LeBron is to a backup on the Knicks. And since the release of *Zero Belly Diet*, more and more evidence keeps proving that point. For example, a study in the journal *Evolution and Human Behavior* found that people who ate more portions of red and orange fruits and vegetables had a more sun-kissed complexion than those who ate less—the result of disease-fighting compounds called carotenoids.

ZERO BELLY FAVORITES  ruby red grapefruit, tart cherries, raspberries, strawberries, blueberries, blackberries, red apples (especially Pink Lady), watermelon, plums, peaches, nectarines

# OLIVE OIL and OTHER HEALTHY FATS
## Vanquish Hunger

Fat does more than just make our food taste good. In fact, the right kinds of fat, like that found in olive oil, nuts, and avocado, can ward off the munchies by regulating hunger hormones. A study published in *Nutrition Journal* found that participants who ate half a fresh avocado with lunch reported a 40 percent decreased desire to eat for hours afterward. And a brand-new study by scientists in India looked at sixty middle-aged men who were at risk for diabetes and heart disease. They gave the two groups similar diets, except that one of these groups got 20 percent of their daily calories from pistachios. The group that ate the pistachios had smaller waists at the end of the study period; their cholesterol score dropped by an average of fifteen points, and their blood sugar numbers improved as well.

**ZERO BELLY FAVORITES**  extra-virgin olive oil, virgin coconut oil, avocados, walnuts, cashews, almonds, almond butter, wild salmon, sardines, ground flaxseed (flax meal), chia seeds

# BEANS, RICE, OATS, and OTHER HEALTHY FIBER
## Turn Off Diabetes Genes

Think of beans as little weight-loss pills, and enjoy them whenever you'd like. One study found that people who ate ¾ cup of beans daily weighed 6.6 pounds less than those who didn't, even though the bean eater consumed, on average, 199 more calories per day. Part of the reason is that fiber—from beans and whole grains—

helps our bodies (okay, actually the bacteria in our bodies) produce a substance called butyrate, which deactivates the genes that cause insulin insensitivity.

One common source of fiber that you won't find in these recipes, however, is wheat. ZERO BELLY isn't strictly a gluten-free program, but all of the recipes in this book use foods that are naturally gluten-free, for a reason: If you have gluten intolerance, then this protein will cause inflammation in your gut. My goal has been to create a plan that will work for everyone. So go ahead and have your Wheaties if you want, but more and more science says that sticking with the ZERO BELLY fiber sources might make more sense: According to a study in the *Annals of Nutrition and Metabolism*, scientists found that having oatmeal (in this case Quaker Oats Quick one-minute oats) for breakfast resulted in greater fullness, lower hunger ratings, and fewer calories eaten at the next meal compared to a serving of ready-to-eat sugared corn flakes, even though the calorie counts of the two breakfasts were identical.

ZERO BELLY FAVORITES   canned black and garbanzo beans, French green lentils, rolled oats, quinoa, brown rice

# Extra Plant Protein
## Boosts Metabolism

One of the unique qualities of ZERO BELLY is its reliance on plant-based proteins. While I'm no vegetarian—not by a long shot!—I also know that relying on dairy-based supplements to boost your protein intake isn't always the best bet for those of us focused on gut health—especially those who suffer from lactose intolerance.

ZERO BELLY FAVORITES   Vega One All-in-One Nutritional Shake, Vega Sport Performance Protein, Sunwarrior Warrior Blend, PlantFusion Protein

# LEAFY GREENS, GREEN TEA, and BRIGHT VEGETABLES
## Stop Inflammation and Turn Off Fat-Storage Genes

A leafy green like Swiss chard is a veritable Swiss Army knife for weight loss. When you eat more greens, you arm your body with high levels of folate, a B vitamin that's been linked to everything from boosting mood to battling cancer. It's also a key that locks down genes linked to insulin resistance and fat-cell formation.

But leafy greens also perform another important function: They help provide you with a healthy, balanced gut. See, it's not enough to just get beneficial bacteria into your body. To make sure the good guys stay healthy and thrive, you need to feed them. And what they really love is something called fructooligosaccharides, or FOS, a type of fiber found in vegetables as well as fruits and grains. But veggies, because of their low caloric load, are probably the healthiest way of all to get these essential nutrients into your belly. FOS has been shown to increase absorption of vitamins and minerals, improve feelings of fullness, and otherwise keep everything running "clean." **ZERO BELLY FAVORITES** kale, spinach, watercress, romaine, carrots, Swiss chard, zucchini, red bell peppers, tomatoes, cucumber, celery, asparagus

# LEAN MEATS and FISH
## Build Muscle and Turn Off Fat-Storage Genes

Maintaining and building muscle is important, especially as we get older. Increased muscle mass means a healthier weight, better fitness, and improved quality of life. But in order to get those benefits, we may need to eat more protein than we currently do. A lot of this can come from plant proteins in our **ZERO BELLY** Drinks. But an extra helping of lean meat might not hurt, either.

Current U.S. recommendations for daily dietary protein are about 0.8 grams per kilogram of body weight, or roughly 62 grams a day for a 170-pound person. A small chicken breast has about 20 grams of protein; so does a serving of ground beef, salmon, or tofu that's about the size of a deck of playing cards. But in a 2015 study in the *American Journal of Physiology—Endocrinology and Metabolism*, researchers found that those who ate twice as much protein as the RDA had greater net protein balance and muscle protein synthesis—in other words, it was easier for them to maintain and build muscle.

**ZERO BELLY FAVORITES**   chicken, lean ground turkey, lean beef, wild salmon, shrimp, scallops, cod, tuna, halibut

# YOUR FAVORITE SPICES
## Turn Off Genes for Inflammation and Weight Gain

At my restaurant White Street, what I get the most compliments on isn't the exotic cocktails, the beefy steaks, or the rich, creamy desserts. It's the little things like vegetable side dishes, soups, and simple meat dishes like roast chicken. And that's because the chefs, like my coauthor Jason Lawless, are masters at the art of mixing and maximizing spices. Jason can make something you've eaten ten thousand times taste like something you've never experienced before.

But herbs, spices, and flavorings do more than add extra pizzazz to your food. From fighting cancer to managing insulin response to fighting inflammation, many popular spices are nutritional stars, and the more you can incorporate them into your daily meals, the better your health and the happier your taste buds.

While most herbs and spices have powerful anti-inflammatory properties, there's a difference between what's in the herb itself and what actually makes its way into your system—what's known as "bioavailability."

To test the actual potency of spices after they've been ingested, researchers at the University of Gainesville, Florida, and at Penn State had subjects eat significant amounts of different spices every day for a week. Then they tested the subjects' blood plasma by dripping it onto inflamed white blood cells. The plasma of subjects who ate cloves, ginger, rosemary, and turmeric were the most potent—in other words, these spices have the highest level of anti-inflammatory impact after ingestion.

That's exciting **ZERO BELLY** news. Cloves, ginger, and rosemary are all essential parts of the *Zero Belly Cookbook* recipes. But turmeric is one of the magical nutrients that's been shown to work directly on our fat genes, turning off the specific genetic mechanism that's responsible for inflammation and obesity. In a 2015 study in the journal *Clinical Nutrition*, researchers gave 117 patients with metabolic syndrome either supplements of curcumin—the active ingredient in turmeric—or a placebo. Over eight weeks, those who received the curcumin saw dramatic reductions in inflammation and fasting blood sugar, another reason why this spice belongs in your pantry.

**ZERO BELLY FAVORITES**   black pepper, turmeric, cinnamon, unsweetened cocoa powder (non-alkalized), cayenne, dried thyme, dried rosemary, dried oregano

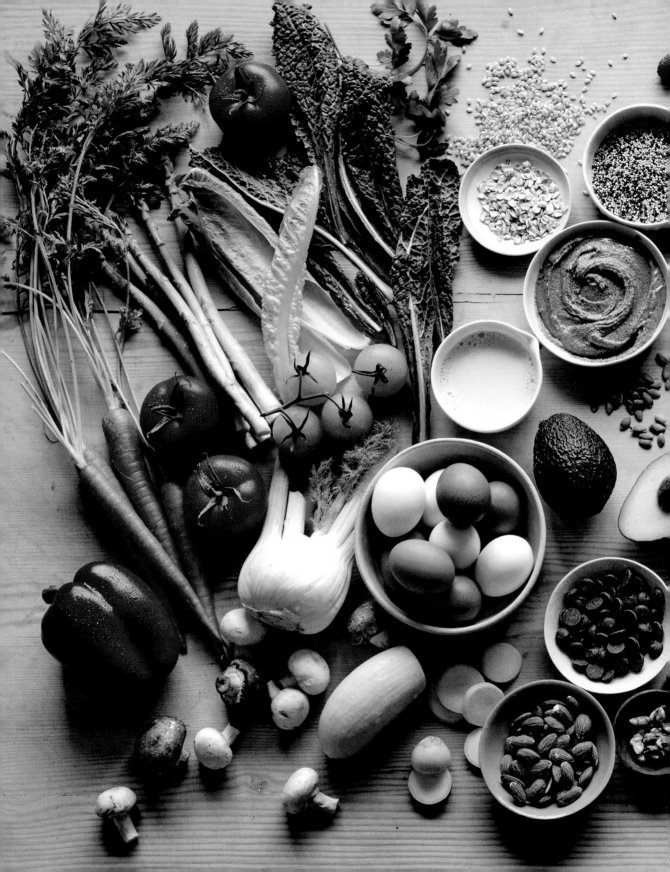

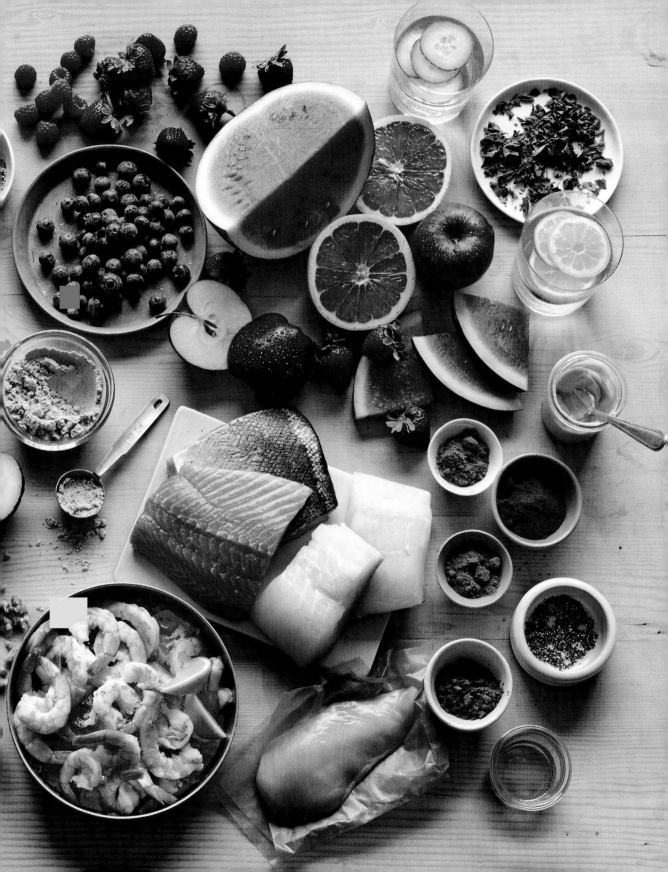

# ZERO BELLY

This comprehensive list of the ingredients is all you'll need to produce the recipes included in this book. Feel free to review the recipes, craft your menu, and adjust your shopping list accordingly!

## OILS & FLAVOR BOOSTERS

- Extra-virgin olive oil
- Virgin coconut oil
- Olive oil cooking spray
- Raw apple cider vinegar
- Canola mayonnaise
- Ketchup
- Dijon mustard
- Pesto
- Tabasco/Sriracha
- Horseradish
- Low sodium Worcestershire sauce
- Low-sodium salsa
- Low-sodium tamari
- Roasted red peppers, packed in water
- Kalamata olives

## SWEETENERS

- Light brown sugar
- Granulated sugar
- Dark chocolate bars or chips (60-70% cocoa solids)
- Unsweetened cocoa powder (non-alkalized)
- Maple syrup
- Raw honey

## SPICE RACK

- Ground cinnamon
- Ground cumin
- Ground ginger
- Garlic powder
- Bay leaves
- Cayenne
- Curry powder
- Paprika
- Rosemary
- Thyme leaves
- Kosher salt
- Black pepper (ground and whole peppercorns)
- Cumin seeds
- Caraway seeds
- Coriander seeds
- Oregano

## NUTS, SEEDS & DRIED FRUITS

- Dried tart cherries
- Assortment of raw, unsalted nuts (walnuts, whole and flaked almonds, pistachios, peanuts, pecans)
- Pepitas
- Natural, no-salt-added peanut butter
- Natural, no-salt-added almond butter
- Flaked coconut (unsweetened)

## ON THE SHELF

- Beans, no salt added (chickpeas, garbanzo, white, kidney, black, pinto)
- Low-sodium broth
- Solid-pack pumpkin
- Diced tomatoes, no-salt added
- Chunk light tuna, packed in water
- Canned salmon
- Unsweetened almond milk (store in fridge after opening)
- Light coconut milk
- Whole coconut milk
- Tea bags (green, white, red, caffeine-free herbal)

## GRAINS

- Gluten-free all-purpose flour
- Almond flour
- Plant-based protein powder (vanilla, chocolate)
- Rolled oats
- Oat flour
- Yellow cornmeal
- Gluten-free breadcrumbs
- Brown rice
- Quinoa

# PANTRY

## IN THE FREEZER

Peeled bananas (halved and stored in BPA-free container)

Assortment of unsweetened berries (blueberries, strawberries, raspberries, mixed berries)

Packages of unsweetened peaches

Shrimp, peeled, deveined, raw

## MEAT, FISH & EGGS

Rotisserie chicken

Skinless, boneless chicken breast

Lean ground turkey (93-99% lean)

Extra-lean grass-fed ground beef (at least 90%)

Atlantic salmon

Smoked salmon

Pacific cod

Swordfish

Halibut

Ahi tuna

Scallops

Eggs

## FRUIT BOWL

Apples (especially Pink Lady or other red varieties; Granny Smith are good also)

Ruby red grapefruits

Red grapes

Melon (watermelon, cantaloupe)

Tart cherries

Berries (strawberries, raspberries, blueberries)

Nectarines/peaches

Oranges

Limes

Lemons

## VEGGIE DRAWER

Red bell pepper

Celery

Spinach

Arugula

Lettuce (romaine, Bibb/Boston, radicchio, iceberg)

Zucchini

Yellow squash

Onions (yellow, white, red)

Mushrooms (cremini, button, shitake)

Eggplant

Carrots

Tomatoes (Roma, grape)

Avocado

English cucumber

Asparagus

Garlic

Idaho/russet potatoes

Sweet potatoes

Fresh ginger

Beets (fresh or pre-roasted—not canned)

## HERB BOX

Parsley

Rosemary

Thyme

Basil

Cilantro

Chives

Mint

## SUPPLEMENTS

Plant-based protein powder blend (Hemp, pea, and rice proteins are all great alternatives to whey. However, a blend is best, as it ensures you're getting a full amino-acid profile. As for flavor, vanilla is recommended for most ZERO BELLY Drink recipes.)

*Recommended brands:*

**Vega One,** All-In-One Shake (Vanilla is classic, but Vanilla Chai also pairs really deliciously with fruit!)

**Natures Plus, Spiru-Tein** (I like Vanilla)

**Sun Warrior, Warrior Blend** (Vanilla or Chocolate)

# ZERO BELLY SPECIAL OCCASION MENUS

Make Every Holiday a Celebration of Healthy and Delicious Foods

## MOTHER'S DAY BRUNCH
Spinach and Onion Strata, page 56
Blueberry Pancakes with Fresh Blueberry Syrup, page 60
Red Fruit Salad, page 205

## FATHER'S DAY DINNER
Mini Crab Cakes "Po Boys" with Sweet Potato Fries, page 122
Steak Frites with Arugula Chimichurri and Asparagus, page 150
Black Forest Cookies, page 206

## CHRISTMAS
Smoked Salmon and Cucumber Rounds with Herbed Mayonnaise, page 178
Perfect Roast Chicken with Roasted Vegetables, page 156
Quinoa "Stuffing" with Dried Cherries and Walnuts, page 252
Chilled Asparagus Salad, page 139
Flourless Chocolate Cake, page 198

## THANKSGIVING
Pumpkin Soup, page 228
Perfect Roast Turkey with Roasted Vegetables, page 157
Quinoa "Stuffing" with Dried Cherries and Walnuts, page 252
No-Crust Pumpkin Pie, page 210

# WARM-WEATHER DINNER PARTY

Avocado with Crab Salad, page 168

Fish and Chips, page 131

Watermelon Wedges with Whipped Coconut Cream, Walnuts, and Mint, page 211

# COOL-WEATHER DINNER PARTY

Mulligatawny Soup, page 143

Black Pepper Shrimp with Creamy Oats, Cherry Tomatoes, and Asparagus, page 128

Apple Crumble, page 190

Whipped Coconut Cream, page 188

# JULY 4

Crudités and Green Goddess Dressing, page 176

Grilled Chicken Kabobs with Whole-Grain Mustard Potato Salad, page 144

Classic Beef Burgers and/or Turkey Burgers with Pesto and Roasted Red Pepper, pages 154 and 135

Chocolate-Dipped Banana Pops, page 201

# COCKTAIL PARTY

Sweet Spiced Nuts, page 164

Artichokes with Garlic Lemon Dipping Sauce, page 174

Smoked Salmon and Cucumber Rounds with Herbed Mayonnaise, page 178

Chicken Satay with Peanut Sauce, page 173

Chocolate Bark, page 186

# THE GAME

BBQ Spiced Nuts, page 164

Buffalo Chicken Skewers, page 180

Mini Crab Cake "Po Boys" with Sweet Potato Fries, page 122

Flourless Chocolate Chip Blondies, page 208

# EASTER

Deviled Eggs, page 168

Marinated Lamb Chops, page 138

Whole Grain Mustard Potato Salad, page 144

Wilted Kale Salad, page 140

Angel Food Cake with Whipped Coconut Cream and Mixed Berries, page 184

# VALENTINE'S DAY

Strawberry Spinach Salad, page 130

Seared Scallops with Roasted Fingerling Potatoes and Red Apple Slaw, page 120

Chocolate-Covered Strawberries, page 209

# BREAKFAST HASH with POACHED EGG

SERVES: 4 | COOK TIME: 15 MINUTES

½ **bunch green asparagus,** white part of stems removed, cut into 1-inch pieces

1 **small yellow squash,** sliced into ¼-inch half-moons

1 **small zucchini,** sliced into ¼-inch half-moons

1 **small onion,** diced

1 **cup white button mushrooms,** quartered

1 **red bell pepper,** diced

1 **tbsp extra-virgin olive oil**

1 **tsp kosher salt**

1 **tsp freshly ground black pepper**

4 **eggs**

3 **tbsp coarsely chopped fresh parsley**

3 **tbsp coarsely chopped fresh chives**

- Preheat the oven to 350°F.

- Combine the asparagus, yellow squash, zucchini, onion, mushrooms, bell pepper, olive oil, salt, and black pepper in a large bowl and mix well. Transfer to a nonstick rimmed baking sheet, and bake in the oven for about 10 minutes or until the vegetables are tender.

- While the vegetables are cooking, poach the eggs (see page 73 for instructions).

- Transfer the cooked vegetables to a bowl with the parsley and chives and mix well.

- Divide the vegetable hash among four bowls, and top each with one poached egg.

**PER SERVING:** 160 calories / 9 g fat / 12 g carb / 4 g fiber / 9 g protein

# ORANGE and WALNUT WAFFLES with SUNKIST SYRUP

SERVES: 4    COOK TIME: 10 MINUTES

2   eggs

1   egg white

1   cup unsweetened almond milk

1   tbsp extra-virgin olive oil

1   tsp vanilla extract

2   cups oat flour

2   tbsp vanilla plant-based protein powder

½   tsp salt

2   tsp baking powder

3   tbsp raw walnuts, toasted in a dry pan over medium heat until fragrant (about 2 minutes) and coarsely chopped

**Zest of 2 oranges**

*Syrup*

2   tbsp maple syrup

1   large orange, peeled, segmented, and chopped

- In a large bowl, whisk together the eggs, egg white, almond milk, olive oil, and vanilla.

- In a separate bowl, mix together the flour, protein powder, salt, and baking powder.

- Combine the wet and dry ingredients in a bowl and mix until smooth.

- Fold in the walnuts and the orange zest.

- Heat a waffle iron according to directions. For four waffles, ladle ¼ cup batter onto the heated waffle iron and cook according to the directions on your waffle iron.

- While the waffles are cooking, combine the syrup and oranges in a bowl.

- Divide the waffles among four plates and top with a spoonful of the citrus syrup.

**PER SERVING (2 waffles):** 322 calories / 13 g fat / 41 g carb / 6 g fiber / 14 g protein

# SPINACH and ONION STRATA

SERVES: 4    COOK TIME: 1 HOUR

1½ tsp **extra-virgin olive oil**

1 **large white onion,** coarsely chopped

2 **cups fresh spinach,** packed

4 **slices gluten-free bread,** cut into ½-inch cubes

3 **whole eggs**

6 **egg whites**

1¼ **cups unsweetened almond milk**

1 **tbsp Zero Belly Sofrito** (page 238)

1 **tsp kosher salt**

½ **tsp freshly ground black pepper**

- Heat a large sauté pan over medium heat. Add the olive oil and onion to the pan and cook until the onion becomes slightly translucent and soft. Add the spinach and cook until wilted. Transfer the cooked vegetables to a colander to remove any excess moisture. Set aside to cool completely.

- Place the cubed bread in the bottom of a large pie dish and top with the spinach and onion mixture.

- In a large bowl, whisk together the eggs, egg whites, almond milk, sofrito, salt, and pepper. Pour over the bread and spinach mixture, cover with plastic wrap, and place the dish in the fridge overnight, or at least 4 hours.

- Preheat the oven to 350°F.

- Remove the plastic wrap from the strata and cook uncovered for 45 minutes or until the eggs are fully cooked.

- Let rest for 5 minutes before slicing. Serve warm.

**PER SERVING:** 249 calories / 11 g fat / 24 g carb / 2 g fiber / 13 g protein

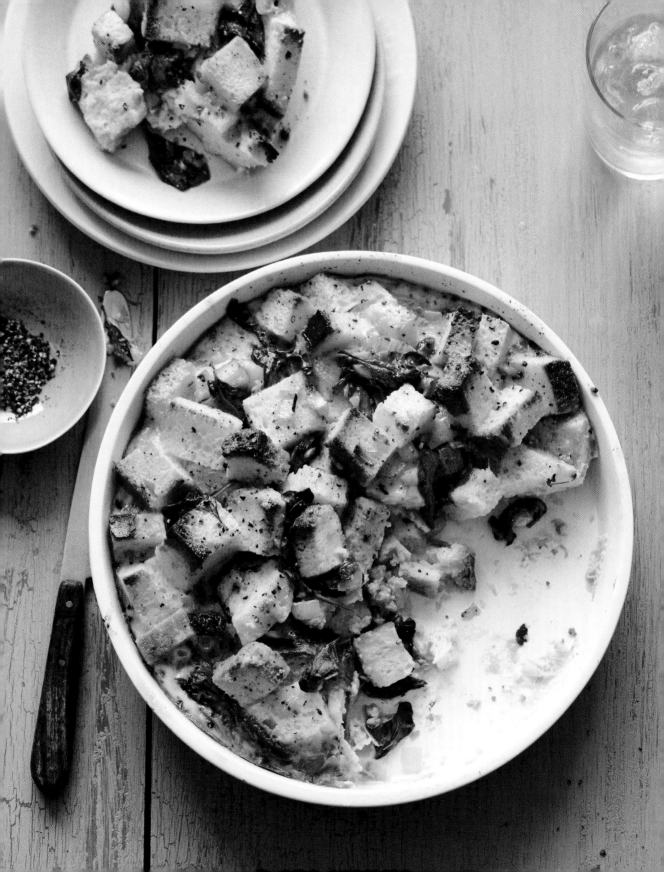

# APPLE PIE MUFFINS

YIELD: 12 MUFFINS    COOK TIME: 30 MINUTES

1½   cups gluten-free all-purpose flour

2   tbsp vanilla plant-based protein powder

¼   cup rolled oats

¼   tsp baking powder

1   tsp ground cinnamon

½   tsp ground nutmeg

2   eggs

¼   cup unsweetened applesauce

¼   cup maple syrup

¼   cup unsweetened almond milk

3   tbsp extra-virgin olive oil

½   tsp vanilla extract

1   red apple, cored and grated (skin on)

¼   cup raw walnuts, toasted in a dry pan over medium heat until fragrant (about 2 minutes) and coarsely chopped

Olive oil spray

- Preheat the oven to 350°F.

- In a large bowl, combine the flour, protein powder, oats, baking powder, cinnamon, and nutmeg.

- In another bowl whisk together the eggs, applesauce, maple syrup, almond milk, olive oil, vanilla, and apple.

- Combine the wet and dry ingredients and mix until just combined. Fold in the walnuts.

- Spray a standard 12-hole muffin tin with olive oil spray. Pour the batter into the prepared muffin pan. Tap the pan on the counter a few times to remove any air bubbles. Bake for 15 to 20 minutes, or until a wooden toothpick inserted in the center of one of the muffins comes out clean.

- Let cool on a wire rack for 15 minutes. Run a knife around the muffins to loosen them and unmold. Serve warm or at room temperature.

**PER MUFFIN:** 133 calories / 7 g fat / 14 g carb / 4 g fiber / 5 g protein

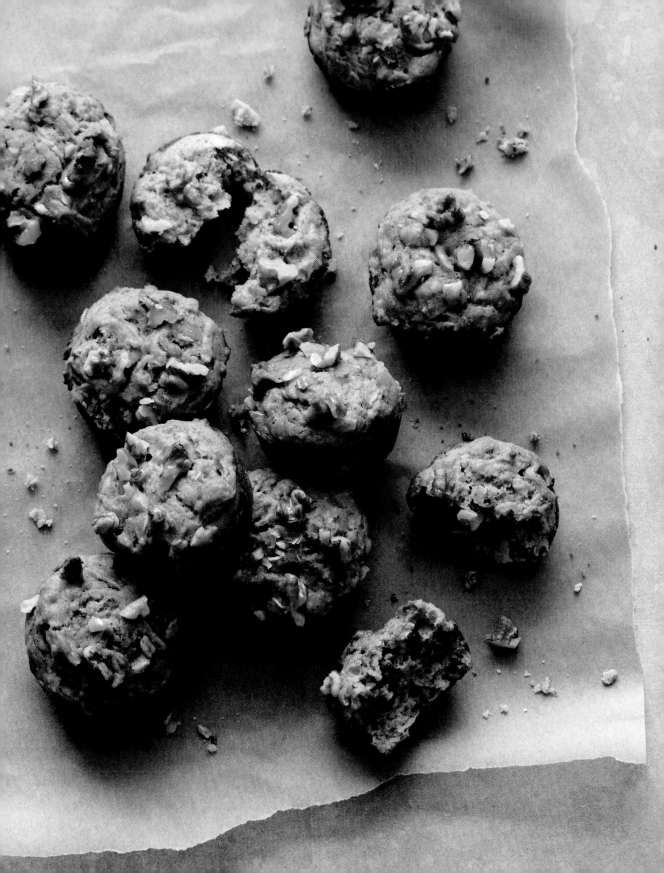

# BLUEBERRY PANCAKES with FRESH BLUEBERRY SYRUP

SERVES: 4    COOK TIME: 10 MINUTES

### Syrup

¼   cup fresh blueberries

2   tbsp maple syrup

2   tbsp water

### Pancakes

2   cups oat flour

1   tbsp baking powder

¼   tsp kosher salt

1   cup unsweetened almond milk

1½  tsp extra-virgin olive oil

1   egg

½   tsp vanilla extract

    Juice of half a lemon

2   egg whites, whipped to soft peaks

    Olive oil spray

½   cup fresh blueberries

- Prepare the syrup. Combine the blueberries, maple syrup, and water in a small saucepan, and place over medium heat. Bring to a low simmer, and cook for 5 minutes, stirring occasionally. Set aside.

- Heat a griddle or a large cast-iron pan over medium heat.

- In a bowl, mix together the oat flour, baking powder, and salt.

- In a separate bowl, whisk together the almond milk, olive oil, egg, vanilla, and lemon juice.

- Combine the wet and dry ingredients and mix until just combined.

- Gently fold in the egg whites.

- Lightly coat the griddle or cast-iron pan with olive oil spray, and use a 2-ounce ladle or a ¼-cup measure to ladle the pancakes onto the pan.

- Cook for about 2 minutes on the first side. Just before flipping, top with a few blueberries. Flip the pancake with a heatproof spatula and cook for 1 to 2 minutes more.

- Repeat with remaining batter for about 12 pancakes total.

- Divide the pancakes among four plates (three per plate) and top with a spoonful of the blueberry syrup.

**PER SERVING (3 pancakes):** 261 calories / 7 g fat / 35 g carb / 7 g fiber / 11 g protein

# BREAKFAST SANDWICH

SERVES: 4    COOK TIME: 5 MINUTES

**4** **slices gluten-free bread,** toasted

**2** **tbsp Zero Belly Mayonnaise** (page 242), or store-bought

**4** **eggs**

**1** **Roma tomato,** sliced

**½** **avocado,** sliced

**4** **Bibb lettuces leaves**

**Salt and freshly ground black pepper to taste**

- Toast the bread until golden brown.

- Spread each slice of toast with 1½ teaspoons mayonnaise and cut each slice in half (8 halves total).

- Cook the eggs sunny-side up or over easy (see page 73 for instructions).

- Lay 1 cooked egg on top of a toast half and top with a slice of tomato, one-quarter of the avocado, and a lettuce leaf. Sprinkle with a pinch of salt and pepper to taste. Top each with another toast half.

- Repeat three times with the remaining ingredients for four sandwiches total. Serve warm.

**PER SERVING:** 213 calories / 9 g fat / 24 g carb / 3 g fiber / 9 g protein

# MEXICAN OMELET with FRESH SALSA

**SERVES: 4 | COOK TIME: 10 MINUTES**

**1 cup canned pinto beans,** drained and rinsed

**Juice of ½ lime**

**Olive oil spray**

**3 eggs**

**5 egg whites**

**½ cup Salsa** (page 245)

**¼ cup Guacamole** (page 243)

- Pulse the pinto beans and lime juice in the bowl of a food processor until it reaches the consistency of refried beans.

- Coat a small nonstick pan with olive oil spray and heat over medium heat.

- Whisk together the eggs and egg whites.

- Add one-quarter of the egg mixture to the pan. Use a spatula to stir, drawing the cooked egg to the center of the pan to let the raw egg slide under.

- When the eggs have all but set, spoon a quarter of the pinto bean mixture down the middle of the omelet. Use the spatula to fold over a third of the egg to cover the mixture, then carefully slide the omelet onto a plate using the spatula to flip it over at the last second to form one fully rolled omelet.

- Top with 2 tablespoons salsa and 1 tablespoon guacamole.

- Repeat three times with the remaining ingredients for four omelets total. Serve immediately.

**PER SERVING:** 197 calories / 8 g fat / 21 g carb / 7 g fiber / 11 g protein

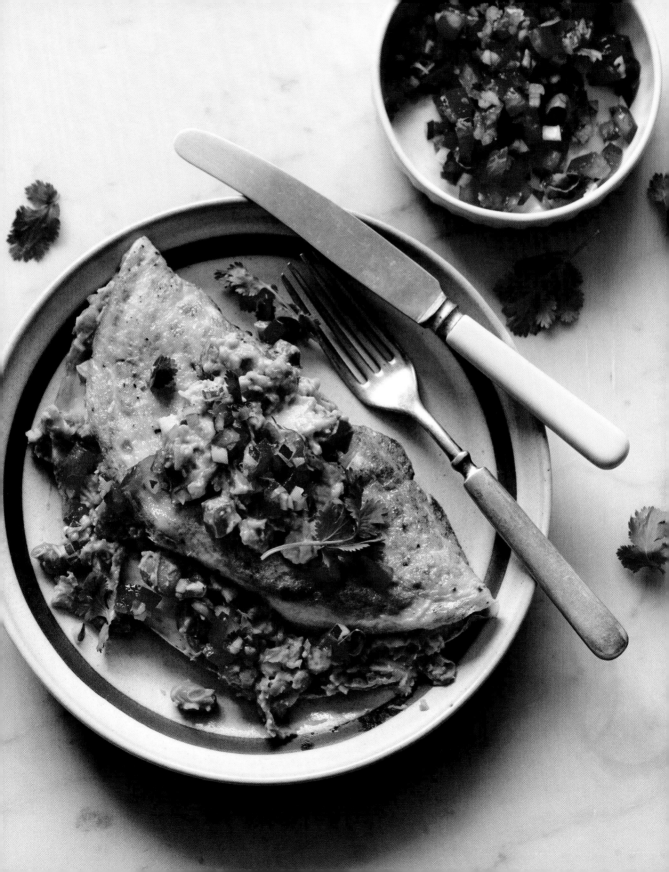

# OATMEAL COMBINATIONS

Alone among cereals, oatmeal packs potent doses of protein as well as fiber. These flavor combinations lift this simple superfood from the mundane to the magnificent.

## PEACH COBBLER (pictured)

**SERVES: 1    COOK TIME: 5 MINUTES**

½ **cup unsweetened almond milk**

½ **cup water**

½ **cup rolled oats**

¼ **tsp ground cinnamon**

½ **cup peaches,** chopped (fresh or frozen and thawed)

1 **tbsp raw flaked almonds**

- Bring the almond milk and water to a boil. Stir in the oats and cook until soft, about 3 minutes. Just before the oats are finished, remove from the heat and stir in the cinnamon, followed by the peaches. Top with the almonds.

**PER SERVING:** 233 calories / 7 g fat / 33 g carb / 5 g fiber / 7 g protein

## APPLE PIE

**SERVES: 1    COOK TIME: 5 MINUTES**

½ **cup unsweetened almond milk**

½ **cup water**

½ **cup rolled oats**

¼ **tsp ground cinnamon**

½ **red apple,** cored and chopped (skin on)

1 **tbsp raw flaked almonds**

- Bring the almond milk and water to a boil. Stir in the oats and cook until soft, about 3 minutes. Just before the oats are finished, remove from the heat and stir in the cinnamon, followed by the apple. Top with the almonds.

**PER SERVING:** 244 calories / 8 g fat / 37 g carb / 6 g fiber / 6 g protein

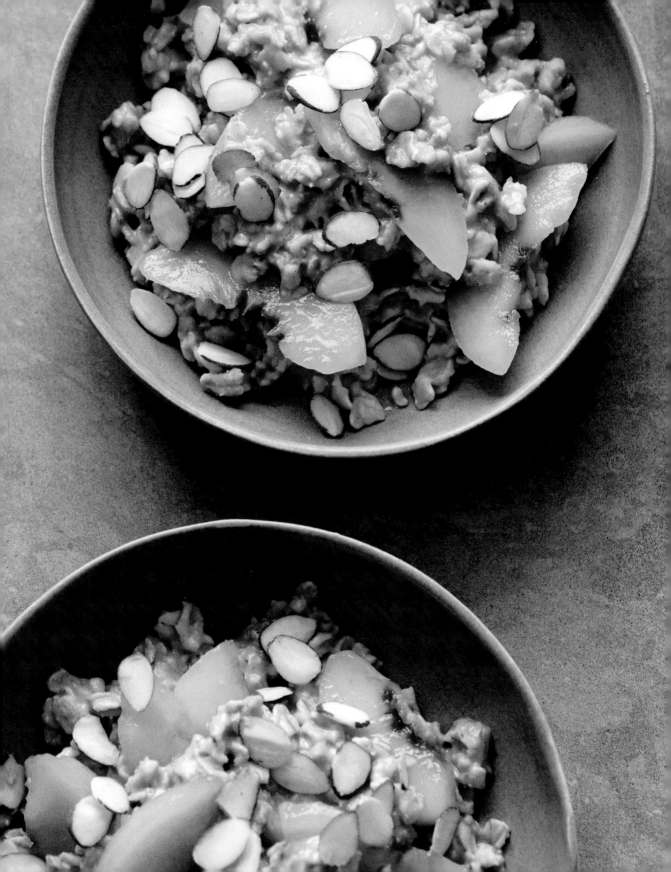

# SUMMER BERRY

**SERVES: 1    COOK TIME: 5 MINUTES**

½   **cup unsweetened almond milk**

½   **cup water**

½   **cup rolled oats**

¼   **tsp ground cinnamon**

½   **cup mixed berries** (fresh or frozen and thawed)

- Bring the almond milk and water to a boil. Stir in the oats and cook until soft, about 3 minutes. Just before the oats are finished, remove from the heat and stir in the cinnamon, followed by the berries.

**PER SERVING:** 200 calories / 5 g fat / 36 g carb / 7 g fiber / 6 g protein

# RASPBERRY ALMOND

**SERVES: 1    COOK TIME: 5 MINUTES**

½   **cup unsweetened almond milk**

½   **cup water**

½   **cup rolled oats**

1   **tbsp vanilla plant-based protein powder mixed with 1 tbsp water until smooth** (optional)

1½   **tsp natural, no-salt-added almond butter**

½   **cup raspberries** (fresh or frozen and thawed)

- Bring the almond milk and water to a boil. Stir in the oats and cook until soft, about 3 minutes. Just before the oats are finished, remove from the heat and stir in the protein powder, if using, followed by the almond butter and raspberries.

**PER SERVING:** 267 calories / 9 g fat / 37 g carb / 9 g fiber / 12 g protein

# BANANA BREAD

½   **cup unsweetened almond milk**

½   **cup water**

½   **cup rolled oats**

¼   **tsp ground cinnamon**

½   **banana,** sliced

1   **tbsp raw pecans,** chopped

- Bring the almond milk and water to a boil. Stir in the oats and cook until soft, about 3 minutes. Just before the oats are finished, remove from the heat and stir in the cinnamon, followed by the banana and pecans.

**PER SERVING:** 268 calories / 9 g fat / 43 g carb / 7 g fiber / 7 g protein

# BLUEBERRY and BLACKBERRY

½   **cup unsweetened almond milk**

½   **cup water**

½   **cup rolled oats**

¼   **tsp vanilla extract**

¼   **tsp ground cinnamon**

¼   **cup blueberries** (fresh or frozen and thawed)

¼   **cup blackberries** (fresh or frozen and thawed)

- Bring the almond milk and water to a boil. Stir in the oats and cook until soft, about 3 minutes. Just before the oats are finished, remove from the heat and stir in the vanilla and cinnamon, followed by the blueberries and blackberries.

**PER SERVING:** 222 calories / 5 g fat / 37 g carb / 7 g fiber / 10 g protein

# PIÑA COLADA

**SERVES: 1  COOK TIME: 5 MINUTES**

¼ **cup light coconut milk**

¾ **cup water**

½ **cup rolled oats**

¼ **cup chopped pineapple** (fresh)

1 **tbsp unsweetened coconut flakes**

1 **tsp raw Manuka honey** (optional)

- Bring the coconut milk and water to a boil. Stir in the oats and cook until soft, about 3 minutes. Just before the oats are finished, remove from the heat and stir in the pineapple. Top with the coconut and drizzle with honey, if desired.

**PER SERVING:** 253 calories / 11 g fat / 34 g carb / 6 g fiber / 6 g protein

# CARROT CAKE

**SERVES: 1  COOK TIME: 5 MINUTES**

½ **cup unsweetened almond milk**

½ **cup water**

½ **cup rolled oats**

⅓ **cup grated carrot**

¼ **banana,** sliced

1 **tsp maple syrup**

¼ **tsp ground cinnamon**

1 **tbsp raw walnuts,** chopped

- Bring the almond milk and water to a boil. Stir in the oats and carrot and cook until soft, about 3 minutes. Just before the oats are finished, remove from the heat and stir in the banana, maple syrup, and cinnamon, followed by the walnuts.

**PER SERVING:** 274 calories / 9 g fat / 35 g carb / 7 g fiber / 7 g protein

# BANANA SPLIT

- ½  **cup unsweetened almond milk**
- ½  **cup water**
- ½  **cup rolled oats**
- 1  **tbsp vanilla plant-based protein powder mixed with 1 tbsp water until smooth** (optional)
- ¼  **banana,** sliced
- ¼  **cup strawberries,** sliced (fresh or frozen and thawed)
- 1  **tbsp semisweet chocolate chips**

- Bring the almond milk and water to a boil. Stir in the oats and cook until soft, about 3 minutes. Just before the oats are finished, remove from the heat and stir in the protein powder, if using, followed by the banana and strawberries. Top with the chocolate chips.

**PER SERVING:** 296 calories / 9 g fat / 47 g carb / 6 g fiber / 11 g protein

# THE EGG MATRIX

Four steps to a protein-packed, delicious breakfast—
for 250 calories or less!

Simple, round, and perfect: There's no food that's as powerful a weapon against belly fat as the humble egg. Eggs deliver the highest level of protein per calorie of any food in the world, and they're also the greatest single source of choline—a B vitamin that turns off the genes associated with belly fat storage. All of that's nice to know, but it won't be top of mind when you tuck into these stunning breakfast treats.

## STEP 1 › How Do You Like Your Eggs?
### Choose a cooking style:

○ Omelet
○ Personal frittata
○ Poached
○ Sunny-Side Up
○ Over Easy
○ Scrambled

**STAT**

Poached, scrambled, over easy—we all have a preference for how we like our eggs cooked, and a study carried out by the British Egg Industry Council suggests our breakfast order may reveal egg-citing clues into our personalities. The survey of more than 1,000 adults paired the following egg preferences and character traits:

**Poached** > Outgoing
**Boiled** > Disorganized
**Fried** > High sex drive
**Scrambled** > Guarded
**Omelet** > Self-disciplined

## STEP 2 › Plan a Flavor Combo

### Start with
**+ Add**
**+ Add**

**EGGS**

**½ CUP CHOPPED VEGGIES**

**BOOSTER** (OPTIONAL)

1 egg
+
2 egg whites

Tomatoes
Celery
Carrots
Red
bell peppers
Green
bell peppers
Spinach
Zucchini
Yellow squash
Eggplant

Roasted beets
Cooked yellow
or sweet potato
Radish
Mushrooms
Onion
1 tbsp olives
Grilled Mixed
Vegetables
(page 255)
Salsa (page 245)

*Antioxidant Boost*
1 cup greens

*Fiber Boost*
2 tbsp
canned beans

*Healthy Fat Boost*
1 tbsp
Guacamole (page 245) or Pesto
(page 244)

*Metabolism Boost*
Pinch of cayenne or dash of hot sauce

*Flavor Boost*
1 tbsp chopped fresh herbs

# Need Some Inspiration? How About...

### Omelets and Frittatas

## GREEN MARKET
+ Tomatoes
+ Asparagus
+ Spinach

## SOUTHWESTERN
+ Red bell peppers
+ Salsa
+ Beans
+ Guacamole (page 243)

## VEGGIE LOVER
+ Mushrooms
+ Red bell peppers
+ Onion
+ Spinach
+ Asparagus

## GREEK
+ Red onion
+ Black olives
+ Tomatoes
+ Spinach

### Egg Scramble

## NEW MEXICAN
+ Roasted green chilies
+ Tomatoes
+ Hot sauce

## NEW YORKER
+ Smoked salmon
+ Scallions

## SUMMERTIME
+ Grilled Mixed Vegetables
  (page 255)
+ Tomatoes
+ Chopped parsley
+ Basil

### Hash (the perfect bed for a poached or sunny-side up egg)

## NEW ENGLAND
+ Roasted beets
+ Roasted potatoes

## INDIAN SUMMER
+ Zucchini
+ Squash
+ Cooked sweet potato
+ Chopped parsley
+ Basil

## GREEN MACHINE
+ Spinach
+ Asparagus
+ Green bell peppers
+ Pesto (page 242)

*Continued* ›

## STEP 3 ▶ Follow the Instructions Below for the Perfect Dish.

### OMELET (individual)

- Whisk the egg and egg whites together in a small bowl.

- Heat a nonstick pan, lightly coated with olive oil spray, over medium heat.

- Cook the filling: Add the chopped vegetables—and optional boosts of beans, extra greens, and spices, and cook until softened, 2 to 3 minutes.

- Transfer this filling to a plate. Pour the whisked eggs into the heated nonstick pan and let cook, undisturbed, for about 30 seconds.

- Using a rubber spatula, push the cooked egg from the sides of the pan to the center. Tilt the pan to gently draw any uncooked egg to the pan.

- When the eggs are still a bit runny, add the filling to one half of the omelet.

- Fold the omelet in half using a spatula and slide the omelet out of the pan to a plate.

- Top with optional boosts of fresh herbs, guacamole, or pesto, if desired.

- Serve immediately.

### FRITTATA (individual)

- Preheat the oven to 350°F, or heat a broiler on medium.

- In an oven-proof pan, follow the instructions for an omelet (individual), but when the egg is halfway set, sprinkle the filling across the entire surface of the egg.

- Remove from the heat and finish in the oven for 5 minutes, or under the broiler for 2 to 3 minutes, until the eggs are set.

- Shake out of the pan onto a plate.

- Top with optional boosts of fresh herbs, guacamole, or pesto, if desired. Serve hot, at room temperature, or chilled.

### SOFT SCRAMBLE

- Whisk together the egg and egg whites with 1 tablespoon unsweetened almond milk.

- Heat a nonstick pan, lightly coated with olive oil spray, over medium heat.

- Add the chopped vegetables—and optional boosts of beans, extra greens, and spices, and cook until softened, 2 to 3 minutes.

- Reduce the heat to low, add the whisked eggs to the pan, turn and fold with a rubber spatula.

- When the eggs are almost cooked through but still runny, remove the pan from the heat to allow for carry-over cooking.

- Top with optional boosts of fresh herbs, guacamole, or pesto if desired.

- Serve immediately.

### HARD SCRAMBLE

- Continue cooking in the pan until firm.

### POACHED EGG and VEGGIE HASH

- Add enough water to come 1 inch up the side of a medium saucepan and bring to a simmer over medium heat.

- Add 1 tablespoon white vinegar.

- Crack the egg into a small bowl.

- Using a large spoon or spatula, swirl the simmering water in the pan to create a "whirlpool," and then carefully drop the egg into the center.

- Repeat with the whites (if using). Leave the eggs to cook, undisturbed, for about 5 minutes.

- Meanwhile, heat a nonstick pan lightly coated with olive oil spray over medium heat.

- Add the chopped vegetables—and optional boosts of beans, extra greens, and spices—and cook until softened, 2 to 3 minutes.

- Turn off the heat and transfer the cooked veggies to a plate.

- Remove the poached egg and whites from the whirlpool with a slotted spoon and serve on top of the veggie hash.

- Top with optional boosts of fresh herbs, guacamole, or pesto, if desired.

- Serve immediately.

### SUNNY-SIDE UP and VEGGIE HASH

- Heat a nonstick pan lightly coated with olive oil spray over medium heat.

- Add the chopped vegetables and optional boosts of beans, extra greens, and spices and cook until softened, 2 to 3 minutes.

- Transfer the cooked veggies to a plate for serving.

- Keep the pan on the stove.

- Crack the egg and egg whites into a small bowl and add directly into the pan. Fry until the edges are golden brown and the egg white is fully cooked.

- Slide the egg and whites onto the veggie hash, and top with optional boosts of fresh herbs, guacamole, or pesto, if desired.

- Serve immediately.

### OVER EASY and VEGGIE HASH

- Follow the instructions for Sunny-Side Up and Veggie Hash.

- When the edges of the fried eggs are golden brown and the egg white is fully cooked, flip the egg with a spatula and cook for another minute; the yolk will still be runny.

- Slide the egg and whites onto the veggie hash and top with optional boosts of fresh herbs, guacamole, or pesto, if desired.

### OVER MEDIUM and VEGGIE HASH

- Cook for 2 minutes more once flipped; the yolk will be semi-soft.

- Serve immediately.

### OVER HARD and VEGGIE HASH

- Cook for 3 minutes more once flipped; the yolk will be hard.

- Serve immediately.

# CHAPTER FOUR

# ZERO BELLY LUNCHES

How to Turn the **ZERO BELLY** Foods into Delicious, Easy-to-Make Meals That Are Ready in Minutes

When people ask me what's so unique about the **ZERO BELLY** meal plan, I tell them this: It involves eating food.

By that I mean real food—food with the power to reverse the fat-gene switches that are triggered by our modern, processed diets and set us back on the path to perfect health.

In 2013, I wrote *Eat It to Beat It,* which looked at the additives in food and how these ingredients were making us fat—by causing inflammation and digestive distress. In fact, studies show that the more processed food you eat, the greater your weight—even if you eat the same number of calories.

Let me repeat that: Eating processed foods instead of real foods will make you gain weight, even if you're eating the same number of calories.

It all goes back to inflammation, and why I built **ZERO BELLY** to calm the fire and turn off the fat-storage genes that processed foods turn on.

# EASY CHICKEN and RICE SOUP

SERVES: 4    COOK TIME: 15 MINUTES

½  **rotisserie chicken**

1  **tbsp extra-virgin olive oil**

½  **cup finely diced onion**

½  **cup finely diced celery**

½  **cup finely diced carrot**

2  **cups low-sodium chicken broth**

3  **cups low-sodium vegetable broth**

1  **tsp kosher salt**

1  **cup cooked Brown Rice** (page 253)

¼  **cup chopped fresh herbs** (your choice)

- Remove the skin from the chicken. Pick the meat, both white and dark, from the carcass and shred. Reserve half of the meat for a future meal.

- Heat the olive oil over medium heat in a 4-quart pot. Add the onion, celery, and carrot and cook until soft, about 5 minutes.

- Add the chicken broth, vegetable broth, and salt to the pot and bring to a boil. Reduce the heat and simmer for 10 minutes more.

- Add the chicken, rice, and fresh herbs and simmer for 5 minutes more. Serve hot.

**PER SERVING:** 225 calories / 10 g fat / 18 g carb / 3 g fiber / 15 g protein

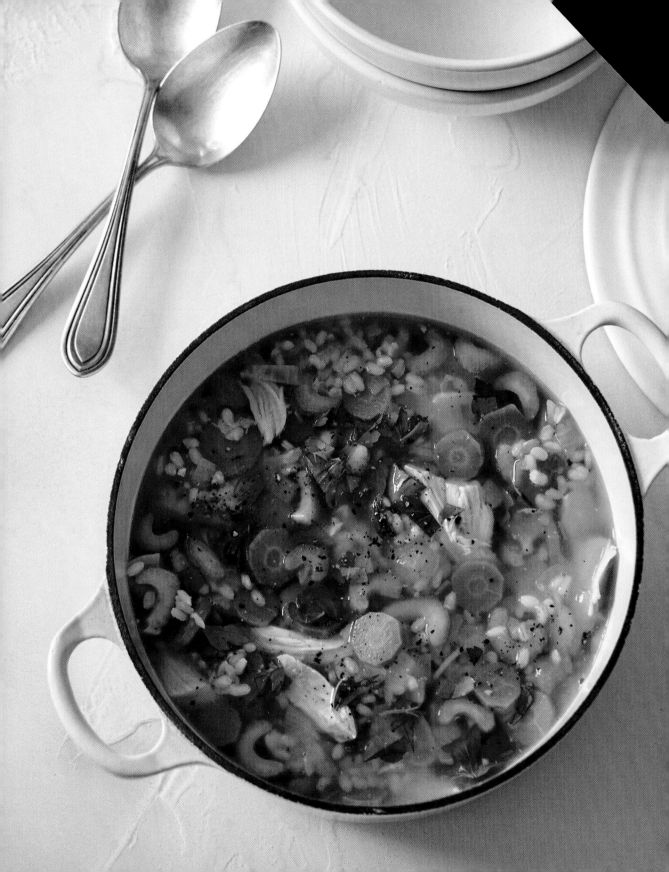

# CURRIED CHICKEN SALAD LETTUCE WRAPS

SERVES: 4    COOK TIME: 25 MINUTES

½  **rotisserie chicken**

¼  **cup Zero Belly Mayonnaise** (page 242), or store-bought

1  **tbsp fresh lemon juice**

2  **tsp curry powder**

3  **tbsp coarsely chopped fresh mint**

3  **tbsp coarsely chopped fresh cilantro**

¼  **cup red grapes,** halved

2  **tbsp raw flaked almonds,** toasted in a dry pan over medium heat until fragrant (about 2 minutes)

⅓  **cup coarsely chopped red onion**

3  **stalks celery,** sliced thin into half-moons

1  **head Bibb lettuce leaves**

- Remove the skin from the chicken. Pick the meat, both white and dark, from the carcass and shred. Reserve half of the meat for a future meal.

- Mix together the mayonnaise, lemon juice, curry powder, mint, and cilantro in a large bowl. Fold in the shredded chicken, grapes, almonds, red onion, and celery.

- Spoon the salad on top of lettuce leaves and divide the wraps among four plates.

 TIP  Save Your Hearts! Use up leftover lettuce hearts in Seared Tuna with Lettuce Heart Salad on page 84.

**PER SERVING:** 251 calories / 13 g fat / 8 g carb / 3 g fiber / 24 g protein

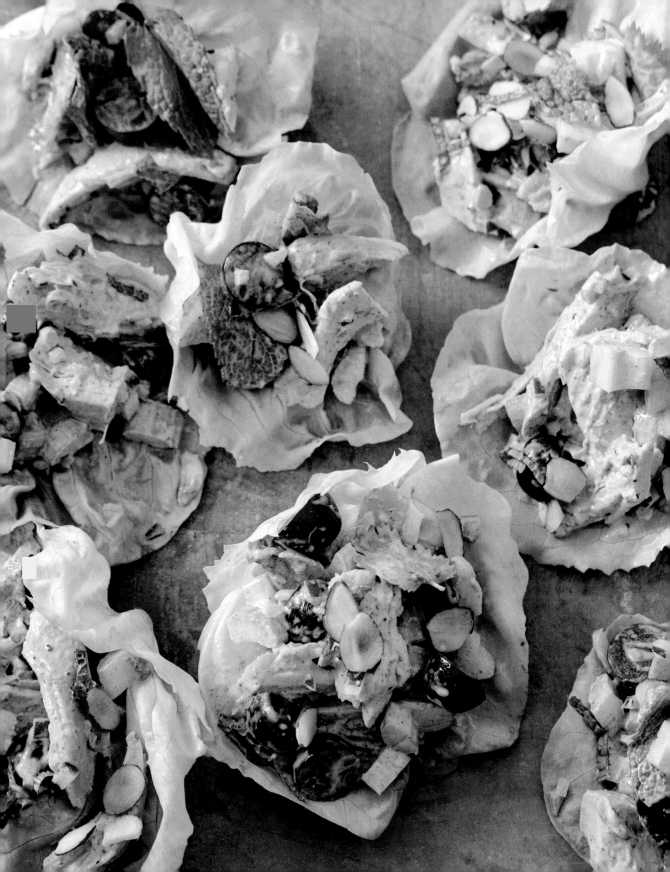

# CHICKEN and BEAN BURRITO

SERVES: 4    COOK TIME: 5 MINUTES

½ **rotisserie chicken**

½ **cup cooked Brown Rice**
(page 253)

½ **cup canned
pinto beans,**
drained and rinsed

4 **gluten-free tortillas**

1 **cup Salsa**
(page 245)

¼ **cup Guacamole**
(page 243)

- Remove the skin from the chicken. Pick the meat, both white and dark, from the carcass and shred. Reserve half of the meat for a future meal.

- Heat the shredded chicken, rice, and pinto beans in the microwave or a small saucepan over medium heat until warm.

- Warm the tortillas in the microwave or in a dry pan over medium heat.

- Divide the chicken mixture among four tortillas and top each with ¼ cup salsa and 1 tablespoon guacamole. Roll up the burritos and serve warm.

**PER SERVING:** 337 calories / 11 g fat / 36 g carb / 7 g fiber / 26 g protein

# TURKEY CLUB

SERVES: 4   COOK TIME: 5 MINUTES

8 slices gluten-free bread

¼ cup Dijon mustard

¾ lb low-sodium organic
deli turkey meat,
thinly sliced

½ avocado,
sliced

1 Roma tomato,
sliced

8 Bibb lettuce leaves

2 tbsp Zero Belly
Mayonnaise
(page 242)

- Toast the bread until golden brown.

- Spread four slices of toasted bread with 1 tablespoon Dijon each. Top each with one-quarter of the turkey and sliced avocado, a slice of tomato, and 1 lettuce leaf.

- Spread the four remaining slices of toast with 1½ teaspoons mayonnaise, and place on top of each of the sandwiches. Slice each sandwich in half and serve.

**PER SERVING:** 305 calories / 10 g fat / 30 g carb / 8 g fiber / 24 g protein

# ENGLISH MUFFIN PIZZAS

SERVES: 4    COOK TIME: 10 MINUTES

| | |
|---|---|
| 2 | **gluten-free English muffins,** split in half |
| ½ | **cup Marinara** (page 241) |
| 12 | **Turkey Meatballs** (page 247), coarsely chopped |
| 1 | **small yellow onion,** thinly sliced |
| 8 | **oz white button mushrooms,** thinly sliced |
| 1 | **tsp dried oregano** (optional) |
| ¼ | **cup fresh basil,** coarsely chopped |
| 2 | **cups packed mixed greens** |
| 1 | **tbsp Zero Belly Vinaigrette** (page 236) |

- Toast the English muffin halves until golden brown.

- Preheat the oven to 350°F.

- Spoon 2 tablespoons marinara on top of each toasted English muffin half for four individual pizzas. Divide the meatballs among the four muffin halves, along with the sliced onion and mushrooms. Sprinkle with oregano, if desired.

- Place the English muffin halves on a rimmed baking sheet. Bake in the oven for 5 to 10 minutes. Garnish with the basil.

- Toss the mixed greens and vinaigrette in a large bowl.

- Divide the mixed greens among four plates and serve with one pizza on each plate.

**PER SERVING:** 309 calories / 10 g fat / 29 g carb / 6 g fiber / 35 g protein

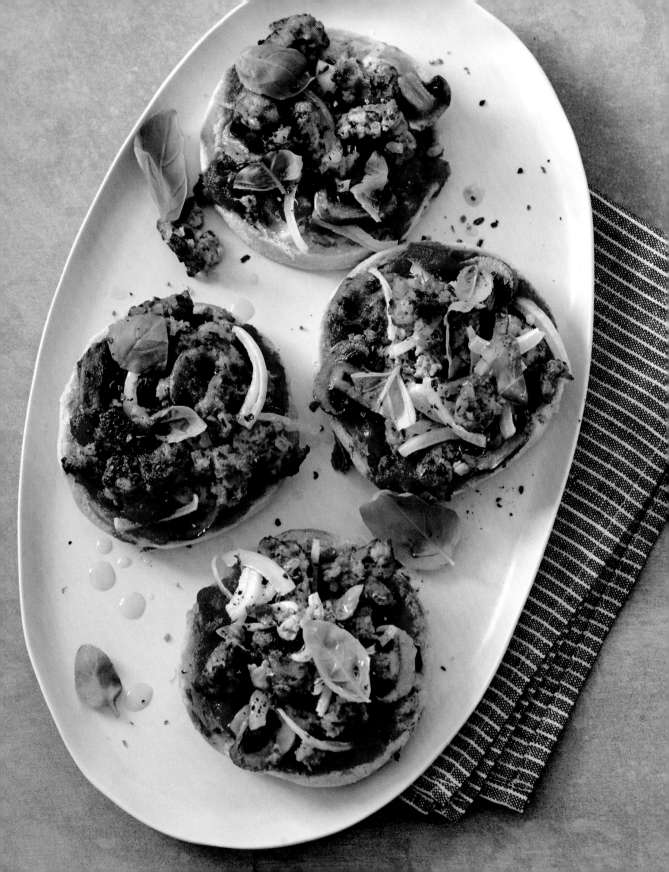

# SEARED TUNA with LETTUCE HEART SALAD

**SERVES: 4** | **COOK TIME: 15 MINUTES**

## Salad

**4** **cups lettuce hearts,** chopped

**¼** **cup fresh blueberries**

**¼** **cup canned garbanzo beans,** drained and rinsed

**1** **red apple,** quartered, seeded, and sliced thin

**¼** **English cucumber,** sliced into half-moons

**2** **tbsp raw walnuts,** toasted in a dry pan over medium heat until fragrant (about 2 minutes) and coarsely chopped

**3** **tbsp Zero Belly Vinaigrette** (page 236)

**1** **lb Seared Tuna** (page 248)

- Combine the salad ingredients in a large bowl. Mix well and divide among four plates.

- Sear the tuna (page 248).

- Top each salad with 4 ounces seared tuna.

**PER SERVING:** 256 calories / 10 g fat / 13 g carb / 4 g fiber / 29 g protein

# GRILLED VEGETABLE and HUMMUS WRAP

SERVES: 4    COOK TIME: 5 MINUTES

2   **cups Grilled Mixed Vegetables** (page 255), sliced

8   **oz Grilled Chicken Breast** (page 246), cubed

2   **tbsp Pesto** (page 242), or store-bought

4   **gluten-free tortillas**

¼   **cup Hummus** (page 244), or store-bought

1   **cup arugula**

- Combine the grilled vegetables, chicken, and pesto in a large bowl. Set aside.

- Warm the tortillas in the microwave or in a dry pan over medium heat.

- Lay the warm tortillas on a clean surface and spread each with 1 tablespoon hummus. Top each with one-quarter of the grilled vegetables and chicken mixture and a handful of arugula.

- Roll and serve warm.

**PER SERVING:** 286 calories / 12 g fat / 34 g carb / 6 g fiber / 18 g protein

# ASIAN SUMMER ROLLS with SHRIMP and SPICY DIPPING SAUCE

**SERVES: 4   COOK TIME: 20 MINUTES**

8   **rice paper sheets**

8   **sprigs fresh cilantro**

8   **fresh mint leaves**

8   **Bibb or Romaine
     lettuce leaves**
     (about 1 head)

½   **large red bell pepper,**
     quartered and thinly
     sliced

½   **large carrot,**
     sliced thin into
     matchsticks

16  **Poached Shrimp**
     (page 250),
     split in half lengthwise

*Dipping Sauce*

¼   **cup Asian Salad
     Dressing**
     (page 236)

1   **tbsp Sriracha hot sauce**

- Dip the rice paper sheets in a bowl of cold water for 5 to 10 seconds, making sure that all sides are wet, until pliable. Shake off the excess water and place on a clean work surface.

- Place a sprig of cilantro and one mint leave in the front third of the rice paper sheet. Then place a lettuce leaf—rolled into a cigar shape—a few red pepper strips, a few carrot matchsticks, and 4 shrimp halves.

- Fold the bottom of the rice paper wrapper over the filling. Holding the whole thing firmly in place, fold the sides of the wrapper in. Then, pressing firmly down to hold the folds in place, roll the entire wrapper up from the bottom to the top as tight as you can.

- Repeat with the remaining ingredients for eight rolls total.

- To prepare the sauce, whisk together the dressing and hot sauce in a small bowl.

- Serve family style with a small bowl of dipping sauce.

**TIP**   Save Your Hearts! Use up leftover lettuce hearts in Seared Tuna with Lettuce Heart Salad on page 84.

**PER SERVING (2 rolls & 1 tbsp sauce):**
230 calories / 6 g fat / 27 g carb / 2 g fiber / 16 g protein

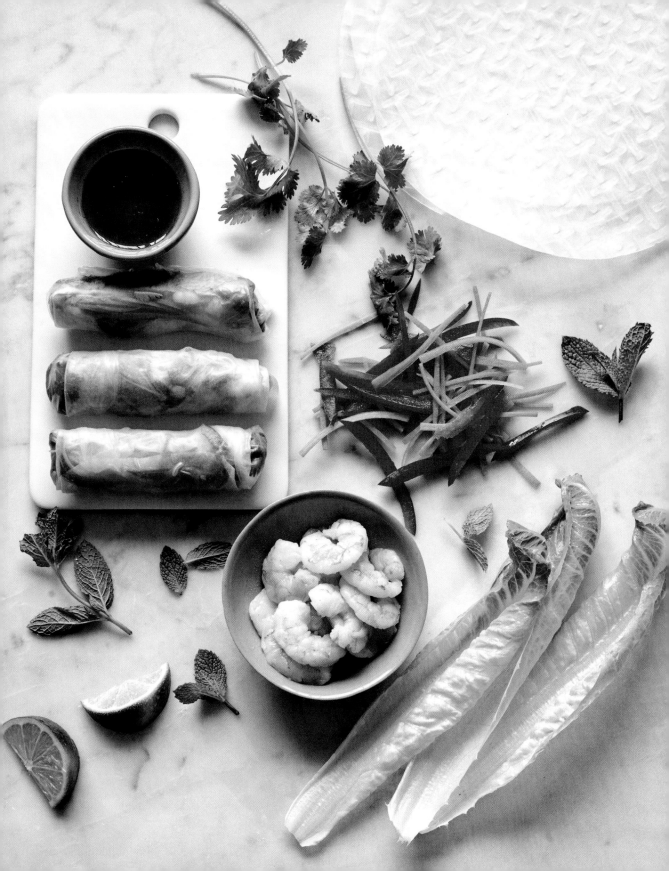

# ASIAN CHICKEN SALAD

SERVES: 4    COOK TIME: 10 MINUTES

½  **store-bought rotisserie chicken**

1  **cup store-bought coleslaw mix**

1  **head romaine lettuce,** chopped

1  **red bell pepper,** seeded, deveined, and thinly sliced

¼  **cup raw slivered almonds,** toasted in a dry pan over medium heat until fragrant (about 2 minutes)

2  **tbsp coarsely chopped fresh mint**

2  **tbsp Asian Salad Dressing** (page 236)

- Remove the skin from the chicken. Pick the meat, both white and dark, from the carcass and shred. Reserve half of the meat for a future meal. Set aside.

- Place all of the remaining ingredients in a large bowl. Mix well and divide among four plates.

- Top each salad with one-quarter of the shredded chicken.

**PER SERVING:** 236 calories / 12 g fat / 13 g carb / 3 g fiber / 20 g protein

# BUFFALO CHICKEN SALAD

SERVES: 4    COOK TIME: 10 MINUTES

½ **store-bought rotisserie chicken**

½ **head iceberg lettuce,** chopped into ½-inch cubes

4 **stalks celery,** sliced thin into half-moons

1 **cup grated carrots**

3 **tbsp raw walnuts,** toasted in a dry pan over medium heat until fragrant (about 2 minutes) and coarsely chopped

1 **tsp celery seeds**

½ **bunch fresh parsley,** coarsely chopped

1 **red apple,** quartered, seeded, and sliced into thin wedges

¼ **cup Red-Hot Buffalo Dressing** (page 237)

- Remove the skin from the chicken. Pick the meat, both white and dark, from the carcass and shred. Reserve half of the meat for a future meal. Set aside.

- Place all of the remaining ingredients in a large bowl. Mix well and divide among four plates.

- Top each salad with one-quarter of the shredded chicken.

**PER SERVING:** 245 calories / 12 g fat / 14 g carb / 4 g fiber / 24 g protein

# MASON JAR SALAD MATRIX

Make a week's worth of to-go lunches in minutes!

Mason jars are great for shaking up dressings and marinades, storing nuts and dried beans, and keeping leftovers fresh. But one of our favorite ways to use the glass containers is for making salads. All the ingredients stay separate until you shake them together in the jar. Always delicious, never soggy, and ever more eco-chic than plastic Tupperware. What's more, these salads last for days in the fridge. Need a delicious, ready-to-go Zero Belly lunch you can toss into your briefcase or purse and take to the office? Look no further.

### What you need:

- One large Mason jar or other BPA-free container
- One large bowl
- Two forks (for tossing and eating!)
- Cup and tablespoon measures
- Your culinary creativity!

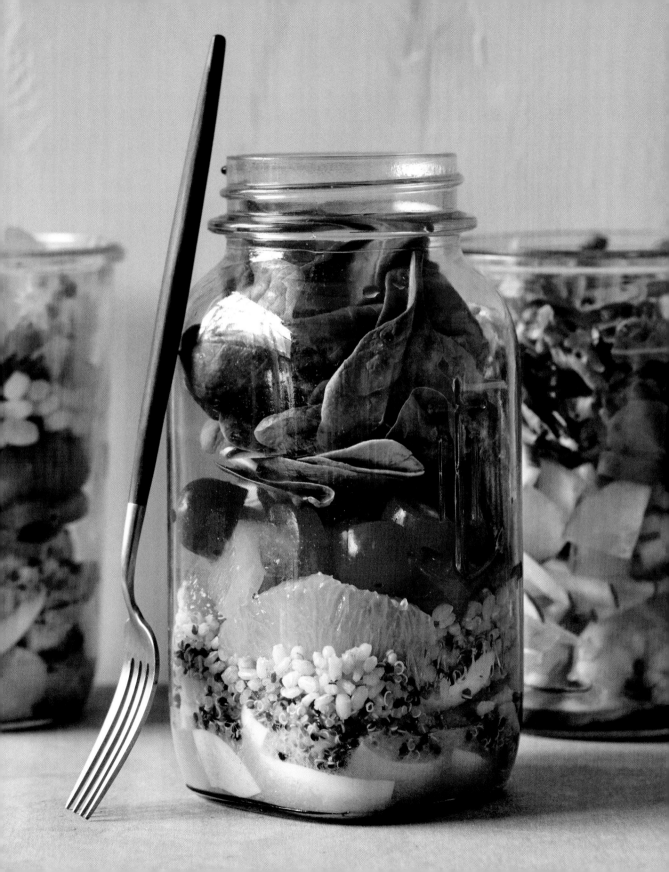

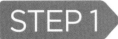 **Plan Your Combo**

Choose up to one portion from each column. You can choose as many ingredients from each column as you like, just stick to the recommended portion. Can't decide between chicken and shrimp? Have 2 ounces of each!

Any way you toss it, the Zero Belly Mason Jar Salad Matrix will serve up a delicious lunch for just 300 calories or less.

## Choose up to one portion from each column

| ½ TBSP DRESSING | 4 OZ COOKED PROTEIN | 1 TBSP HEALTHY FAT | ¼ CUP FIBER, OR FIBROUS VEGETABLE | ½ CUP CHOPPED, BRIGHTLY COLORED VEGETABLES OR FRUIT | 2 CUPS GREENS | FREE EXTRAS |
|---|---|---|---|---|---|---|
| Zero Belly Vinaigrette (page 236) | Grilled Chicken Breast (page 246) | Guacamole (page 243) | Garbanzo beans | English cucumber | Romaine | 1 cup greens |
| Red-Hot Buffalo Dressing (page 237) | Poached Shrimp (page 250) | Zero Belly Mayonnaise (page 242) | Kidney beans | Grape tomatoes | Baby spinach | Fresh herbs |
| Asian Salad Dressing (page 236) | Oven-Roasted White Fish (page 248) | Walnuts | Black beans | Celery | Mixed greens | Spices |
| Italian Dressing (page 237) | Rotisserie chicken (skin removed) | Pistachios | Cannellini beans | Carrots | Iceberg | Pepperoncini |
| Lemon juice | Hard-boiled egg (1 egg + 1 white) | Almonds | Pinto beans | Bell peppers | Watercress | Pickles |
| | Chunk light tuna, packed in water | Pumpkin seeds | Lima beans | Beets | Arugula | |
| | Smoked salmon | Sunflower seeds | Peas | Radish | Radicchio | |
| | Low-sodium deli meat | Olives | Corn | Mushrooms | Bibb lettuce | |
| | Seared Tuna (page 248) | Anchovies | Brown Rice (page 253) | Red onion | Watercress | |
| | Green Lentils (page 254) (½ cup) | | Quinoa (page 251) | Red apple slices | | |
| | | | Gluten-free pasta | Salsa (page 245) | | |
| | | | Sweet Potato Fries (page 122) | Strawberries | | |
| | | | Grilled Mixed Vegetables (page 255) | Grapes | | |
| | | | | Grapefruit segments | | |
| | | | | Orange segments | | |
| | | | | Blueberries | | |
| | | | | 2 tbsp dried tart cherries | | |

## STEP 2 ▸ Build Your Salad

Dressing goes in first — ½ tablespoon. (This guarantees that your salad ingredients don't get soggy.)

Add 4 oz cooked protein.

Add 1 tablespoon healthy fat.

Add ¼ cup fiber or fibrous vegetable.

Add ½ cup chopped low-starch vegetable or fruit.

Add 2 cups greens.

Add FREE extras!

## STEP 3 ▸ Enjoy Your Salad

When you're ready to eat, empty your Mason jar salad into a large bowl and toss. Enjoy!

# Need some inspiration? How about . . .

## CONFETTI
+ Zero Belly Vinaigrette (page 236)
+ Chunk light tuna, packed in water
+ Guacamole (page 243)
+ Kidney beans
+ Corn
+ Cucumber
+ Romaine

## CAESAR
+ Lemon juice
+ Zero Belly Mayonnaise (page 242)
+ Oven-Roasted White Fish (page 248)
+ Anchovies
+ Red onion
+ Carrots
+ Romaine

## CHEF'S
+ Zero Belly Vinaigrette (page 236)
+ Grilled Chicken Breast (page 246)
+ Hard-boiled egg whites
+ Kidney beans

+ Grape tomatoes
+ Cucumber
+ Beets
+ Mixed greens

## LEAN GRAINS
+ Zero Belly Vinaigrette (page 236)
+ Hard-boiled egg
+ Hard-boiled egg whites
+ Quinoa (page 251)
+ Brown Rice (page 253)
+ Citrus segments
+ Grape tomatoes
+ Baby spinach

## SKINNY COBB
+ Zero Belly Vinaigrette (page 236)
+ Grilled Chicken Breast (page 246)
+ Hard-boiled egg whites
+ Guacamole (page 243)
+ Cucumber
+ Grape tomatoes

+ Corn
+ Romaine

## SHREDDED
+ Zero Belly Vinaigrette (page 236)
+ Rotisserie chicken
+ Green beans
+ Corn
+ Grape tomatoes
+ Cucumber
+ Romaine

## ITALIAN
+ Italian Dressing (page 237)
+ Turkey Meatballs (page 247)
+ Black olives
+ Grilled Mixed Vegetables (page 255)
+ Romaine
+ Iceberg
+ Handful of chopped basil

## GARDEN
+ Lemon juice
+ Green Lentils (page 254)

+ Almonds
+ Grape tomatoes
+ Red onion
+ Pepperoncini
+ Mixed greens

## WALDORF
+ Zero Belly Mayonnaise (page 242)
+ Hard-boiled egg
+ Hard-boiled egg whites
+ Walnuts
+ Red apple
+ Celery
+ Dried tart cherries
+ Mixed greens

## ASIAN
+ Asian Salad Dressing (page 236)
+ Poached Shrimp (page 250)
+ Avocado
+ Red bell peppers
+ Radish
+ Cucumber
+ Watercress
+ Arugula
+ Radicchio

# SHRIMP and SNOW PEA SALAD

SERVES: 4    COOK TIME: 10 MINUTES

¾ **lb snow peas**

1 **lb Poached Shrimp**
(page 250)

5 **radishes,**
thinly sliced

¼ **large red onion,**
thinly sliced

1 **large red bell pepper,**
thinly sliced

2 **tbsp coarsely chopped**
**fresh mint**

2 **tbsp coarsely chopped**
**fresh cilantro**

3 **tbsp Asian Salad**
**Dressing** (page 236)

- To blanch the snow peas, bring a medium pot of water to a boil. Fill a large bowl with ice and cold water. Place the snow peas in the boiling water for about 30 seconds, or until tender. Use a large slotted spoon to transfer the snow peas directly into the ice water to cool completely. Once cool, take the snow peas out of the water and place them on a plate lined with paper towels to dry.

- Combine the blanched snow peas and all of the remaining ingredients in a large bowl. Mix well and divide among four plates.

**PER SERVING:** 248 calories / 5 g fat / 18 g carb / 2 g fiber / 25 g protein

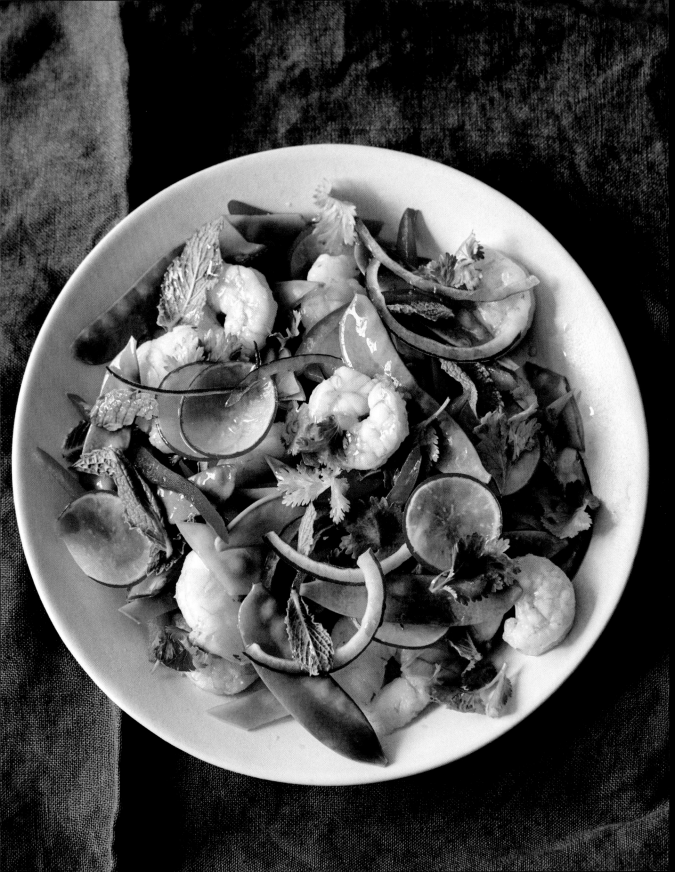

# TURKEY MEATBALL HEROES with ONIONS and PEPPERS

SERVES: 4    COOK TIME: 20 MINUTES

4 **gluten-free hot dog buns**

1½ **tsp extra-virgin olive oil**

½ **large white onion,** sliced thin

1 **large red bell pepper,** quartered and sliced thin

1 **cup Marinara** (page 241)

20 **Turkey Meatballs** (page 247)

- Toast the hot dog buns until golden brown.

- Heat the olive oil in a large sauté pan over medium heat and sauté the onion and bell pepper until tender.

- Add the tomato sauce and the cooked meatballs. Bring to a simmer and cook over low heat for about 5 minutes, stirring occasionally.

- Divide the meatball, onion, and pepper mixture among the four toasted hotdog buns. Serve immediately.

**PER SERVING:** 460 calories / 15 g fat / 37 g carb / 6 g fiber / 23 g protein

# TUNA NIÇOISE SALAD

SERVES: 4    COOK TIME: 15 MINUTES

¼ **lb green beans,** trimmed

½ **lb mixed greens**

¼ **cup cherry tomatoes,** halved

¼ **cup black olives,** halved

½ **bunch fresh parsley,** coarsely chopped

½ **cup canned chickpeas,** drained and rinsed

¼ **cup Zero Belly Vinaigrette** (page 236)

4 **hard-boiled eggs,** * quartered lengthwise

16 **oz chunk light tuna,** packed in water and drained

- To blanch the green beans, bring a medium pot of water to a boil. Fill a large bowl with ice and cold water. Place the beans in the boiling water for about 30 seconds, or until tender. Use a large slotted spoon to transfer the beans directly into the ice water to cool completely. Once cool, take the beans out of the water and place on a plate lined with paper towels to dry.

- In a large bowl, combine the blanched beans, mixed greens, cherry tomatoes, black olives, parsley, chickpeas, and vinaigrette. Mix well and divide among four plates. Top each plate with two quarters of hard-boiled egg and 4 ounces tuna.

See page 250 for a how-to on hard-boiling eggs.

**PER SERVING:** 359 calories / 17 g fat / 14 g carbs / 4 g fiber / 39 g protein

# OVEN-ROASTED COD with TOMATO, QUINOA, and CUCUMBER

**SERVES: 4   COOK TIME: N/A**

*Salad*

2 **cups Quinoa**
(page 251), cooled to
room temperature

2 **tbsp Zero Belly
Vinaigrette** (page 236)

½ **avocado,**
diced

1 **cup packed baby
spinach**

1 **cup cherry tomatoes,**
sliced in half

½ **English cucumber,**
cut in half lengthwise,
then sliced into
half-moons

1 **lb oven-roasted
Pacific cod**
(see Oven-Roasted
White Fish recipe,
page 248)

- Combine the salad ingredients in a large bowl. Mix well and divide among four plates.

- Top each with 4 ounces of oven-roasted cod.

**PER SERVING:** 358 calories / 13 g fat / 24 g carb / 5 g fiber / 35 g protein

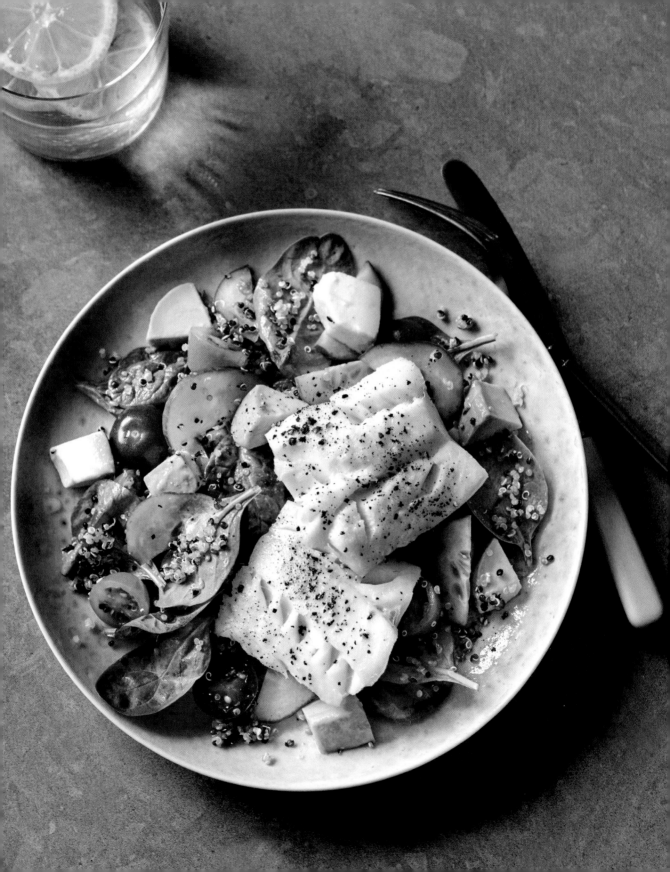

# TUNA and LENTIL SALAD

SERVES: 4 | COOK TIME: N/A

## Salad

- **1 cup Green Lentils** (page 254)
- **½ cup cherry tomatoes,** halved
- **½ avocado,** diced
- **2 cups packed baby spinach,** coarsely chopped
- **2 tbsp Zero Belly Vinaigrette** (page 236)
- **½ bunch fresh parsley,** coarsely chopped
- **½ small red onion,** finely diced
- **¼ tsp salt**

- **1 16-oz chunk light canned tuna,** packed in water, drained

- Combine the salad ingredients in a large bowl. Mix well and divide among four plates.

- Top each with 4 ounces of tuna.

**PER SERVING:** 251 calories / 10 g fat / 15 g carbs / 6 g fiber / 27 g protein

# GRILLED VEGETABLE TARTLETS with CORNMEAL CRUST

**SERVES: 4** | **COOK TIME: 40 MINUTES**

## Crust

- **1 cup fine yellow cornmeal**
- **⅓ cup oat flour**
- **½ tsp salt**
- **3 tbsp cold butter,** cut into small pieces
- **1 egg**
- **1 tbsp extra-virgin olive oil**
- **1 tbsp cold water**

## Filling

- **1 cup Grilled Mixed Vegetables** (page 255), chopped
- **¼ cup cherry tomatoes,** quartered
- **3 tbsp Pesto** (page 242)
- **3 tbsp black olives,** pits removed and coarsely chopped

- **¼ cup coarsely chopped fresh basil** (optional)

- Preheat the oven to 350°F.

- Combine cornmeal, oat flour, salt, butter, egg, and olive oil in the bowl of a food processor and pulse to combine.

- Add the water and pulse until the mixture forms a loose dough. Remove the dough from the processor and press into the bottom and up the sides of four 3-inch individual tart shells (or one large one).

- Bake the shells for about 10 minutes or until the crust is lightly golden brown, and transfer them to a cooling rack to cool slightly. Leave the oven on.

- Combine filling ingredients in a large bowl and divide them among the four cooked tart shells.

- Bake the tarts for 10 minutes more.

- Garnish with the chopped basil. Serve hot or at room temperature.

**PER SERVING:** 250 calories / 15 g fat / 26 g carb / 7 g fiber / 6 g protein

# SEARED TUNA with SHAVED FENNEL, GRAPEFRUIT, and ARUGULA

**SERVES: 4** | **COOK TIME: 15 MINUTES**

*Salad*

1 **fennel bulb,** thinly sliced into half-moons

3 **cups packed arugula**

1 **large ruby red grapefruit,** segmented

¼ **cup coarsely chopped fresh parsley**

3 **tbsp Zero Belly Vinaigrette** (page 236)

1 **lb Seared Tuna (page 248)**

- Combine the salad ingredients in a large bowl. Mix well and divide among four plates.

- Sear the tuna (page 248).

- Top each with 4 ounces of seared, sliced tuna.

**PER SERVING:** 231 calories / 8 g fat / 11 g carb / 3 g fiber / 29 g protein

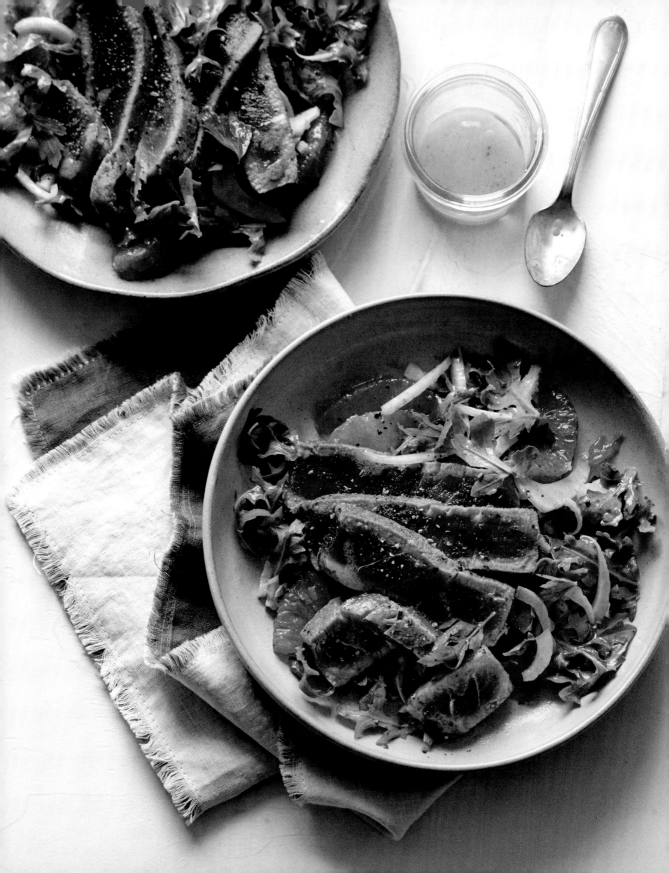

# CHAPTER FIVE

# ZERO BELLY TEST-PANEL FAVORITES

These Pioneers Were Among the First to Experience the Power of **ZERO BELLY**, and Their Incredible Results Inspired a Whole New Collection of Amazing Recipes

'**ve always been blessed** with the greatest family a man could ever ask for. But in the last few years, it's grown quite a bit. By about 1,000 people, in fact.

I call the fans on Facebook's Zero Belly Way of Life my family because they do everything a family should do: support one another, teach one another, step in when they see that one of their own needs a helping hand.

Many of the test panelists who first tried ZERO BELLY have become mentors and coaches for new people just starting the program for the first time. People like June Caron, who lost 26 pounds on the program, and dropped from a size 12 to a size 7. More important, she's kept that weight off, and helped many others do the same. I just had to include a recipe from her, an amazing salmon dish that squeezes six of the ZERO BELLY Foods into one meal! (It's on page 108.) Or Isabel Fiolek, another original ZERO BELLY test panelist who dropped two dress sizes in just six weeks, and has kept that weight off for more than a year. Izzy's White Chicken Chili is on page 106.

What makes ZERO BELLY so much fun is that it's based on real, easy-to-cook foods that people love. I hope you'll experiment with the ZERO BELLY Foods and create your own family recipes. Who knows, you may hand some down to your grandkids. A lifetime of good health: That's a pretty good legacy to leave behind!

# IZZY'S WHITE CHICKEN CHILI

SERVES: 8    COOK TIME: 45 MINUTES

*This chili is well liked by everyone who tries it. I'm frequently asked to share the recipe, and I know from there it has been shared around the world! Low in calories, high in nutrients, and bursting with flavor—what's not to like!*

**—ISABEL FIOLEK, LEESBURG, VA**

1   tbsp extra-virgin olive oil

2   cups onion, chopped

2   cloves garlic, minced

1   tbsp ground cumin

1   tsp dried oregano

1   tsp cayenne pepper (or to taste)

¼   tsp kosher salt

2   4-oz cans green chilies, drained (can substitute with jalapeños)

1   2-lb rotisserie chicken, skin removed, white and dark meat cubed

1   15-oz can cannellini beans, rinsed and drained

3   14-oz cans low-sodium chicken broth

- Heat the olive oil in a large Dutch oven over medium heat.

- Sauté the onion until softened. Add the garlic and sauté for 1 minute. Add the cumin, oregano, cayenne, and salt and cook for 1 minute more.

- Add the chilies, chicken, beans, and stock. Bring to a boil, then reduce the heat and simmer for 40 minutes to blend the flavors.

**PER SERVING:** 321 calories / 5 g fat / 13 g carb / 2 g fiber / 28 g protein

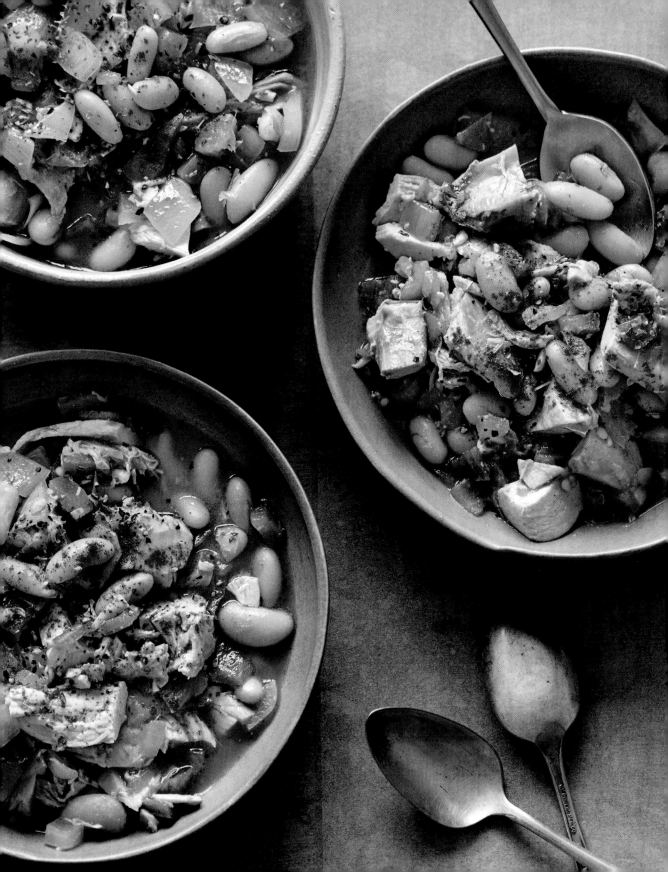

# JUNE'S SALMON MUFFIN PATTIES

SERVES: 6    COOK TIME: 20 MINUTES

*This recipe is very easy and flexible and freezes well for quick future meals. Plus, it's perfectly customizable! You can sub whatever veggies you have on hand, swap tuna for salmon, quinoa for whole oats, and make it your own with your favorite spices and herbs. I've made it dozens of ways, and it always comes out great.*

— JUNE CARON, NORTH OXFORD, MA

¼   **cup unsweetened almond milk**

¾   **cup rolled oats**

1   **small onion,** quartered

½   **red bell pepper,** diced

1   **stalk celery,** coarsely chopped

⅛   **cup packed fresh parsley** (or other fresh herb)

1   **egg,** lightly beaten

1   **14¾-oz can pink or red salmon,** drained

1   **tbsp fresh lemon juice**

¼   **tsp hot sauce**

1   **tsp whole-grain Dijon mustard**

½   **tsp kosher salt**

   **Olive oil spray**

3   **cups packed baby spinach**

1   **tbsp Zero Belly Vinaigrette** (page 236)

- Preheat the oven to 350°F.

- Pour the almond milk over the oats and let soak 5 to 10 minutes while preparing the remaining ingredients.

- In the bowl of a food processor, combine the onion, red pepper, celery, and parsley. Pulse until chopped fine.

- In a large bowl, combine the soaked oats, processed vegetables and herbs, egg, salmon, lemon juice, hot sauce, mustard, and salt. Mix until blended. The mixture will be moist.

- Spray a standard 12-hole muffin tin with olive oil spray and divide the mixture evenly among all twelve cups.

- Bake for 15 to 20 minutes, until the tops are golden and the muffins are firm to the touch.

- Toss the spinach and vinaigrette. Divide the salad among six plates and serve with two muffins.

**PER SERVING (2 muffins):** 143 calories / 6 g fat / 6 g carb / 2 g fiber / 16 g protein

# JULISSA'S EASY TOMATILLO BEEF STEW

SERVES: 4    COOK TIME: 4 TO 8 HOURS

*This recipe is based on a dish my paternal grandmother used to make. She was half-Chinese and half-Mexican and was a wonderful cook. She used to make Colas del Diablo (Devil's Tails), which were tomatillos fried with either pork or beef and served on corn tortillas. This healthier, Zero Belly–friendly version brings my family and me all the flavor and memories without the extra fat.*

— JULISSA LOZA, DESERT HOT SPRINGS, CA

1   **lb stew beef,** cut into 2-inch cubes

1   **large green bell pepper,** chopped into 1-inch chunks

½   **medium onion,** coarsely chopped

10   **tomatillos,** quartered

1   **clove garlic,** minced

½   **cup water**

½   **tsp kosher salt**

½   **tsp freshly ground black pepper**

- Line a slow cooker with a slow cooker bag and combine all of the ingredients.

- Cook on high for 4 hours or on low for 8 hours. The beef will be tender when done and will fall apart with a fork.

**PER SERVING:** 245 calories / 13 g fat / 11 g carb / 3 g fiber / 24 g protein

# BILL'S CHICKEN TACOS

**SERVES: 4    COOK TIME: 20 MINUTES**

*I used to make this meal way before beginning the Zero Belly diet, and it is one of the few meals that made it to the other side! Of course, I did have to remove the loads of cheese, sour cream, and flour tortillas that were packing pounds on me, but I don't miss them one bit! Making and sharing this dish is a delicious reminder that I can still eat the foods I love while keeping myself and my family healthy.*

— BILL GRIESAU, ROCKY HILL, CT

1    tbsp extra-virgin olive oil

1    lb skinless, boneless chicken breasts

Kosher salt and freshly ground black pepper

1    small yellow onion, coarsely chopped

1    medium red bell pepper, coarsely chopped

1    15-oz can black beans, drained and rinsed

1    tsp ground cumin

1    tsp garlic powder

8    small corn tortillas

8    tbsp Salsa (page 245), or store-bought

½    avocado, sliced

¼    cup chopped fresh cilantro for garnish (optional)

- Heat 1½ teaspoons of olive oil in a nonstick pan over medium heat.

- Season the chicken breasts on both sides with a pinch of salt and black pepper and add to the heated pan. Cook for 4 to 6 minutes, flip, and cook for 4 to 6 minutes more.

- Transfer the chicken to a chopping board to cool slightly.

- In the same pan, and over medium heat, add the remaining 1½ teaspoons olive oil, the onion, and the bell pepper. Cook until soft, 2 to 3 minutes. Add the black beans, cumin, and garlic powder to the pan. Season with a pinch of salt and black pepper. Cook until heated through, about 2 minutes.

- Meanwhile, slice or dice the chicken into bite-size pieces.

- Warm the tortillas in the microwave or in a dry pan over medium heat.

- Place two warm tortillas on each of four plates and top with one-quarter of the chicken, veggies, and bean mixture, 2 tablespoons salsa, and a few avocado slices.

- Garnish with cilantro, if desired.

**PER SERVING:** 222 calories / 8 g fat / 19 g carb / 2 g fiber / 19 g protein

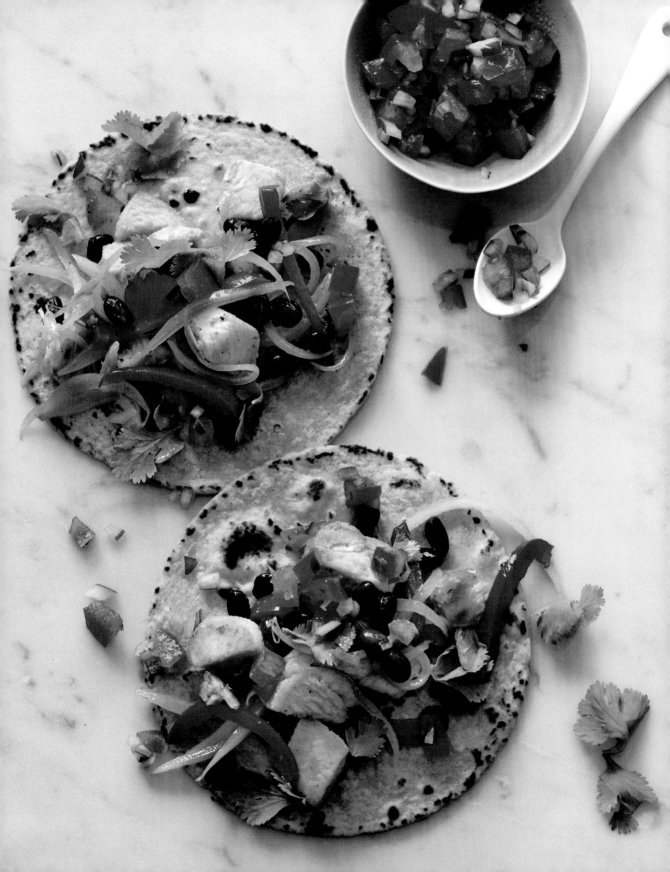

# NICOLETTE'S ONE-POT CHICKEN DINNER

SERVES: 4    COOK TIME: 30 MINUTES

*I've fallen in love with creating new healthy recipes since starting Zero Belly diet and familiarizing myself with the nine super food groups. I decided to create this dish since it includes all three of my favorite Zero Belly ingredients: chicken, mushrooms, and kale. This immediately became a family favorite. And the best part? There is only one pan to clean!*

**— NICOLETTE MARSHALL, FOUNTAIN VALLEY, CA**

- 4 cups Lacinato kale
- 1 tsp smoked paprika
- 1 tsp garlic powder
- 1 tsp ground cumin
- Salt and freshly ground black pepper to taste
- 4 4-oz skinless, boneless chicken breasts (or 1 lb, divided into four portions)
- 1 tsp extra-virgin olive oil
- ½ tbsp virgin coconut oil
- 2 cups cremini mushrooms, sliced
- ½ yellow onion, thinly sliced
- ¼ cup sherry or white wine

**PER SERVING:** 268 calories / 7 g fat / 10 g carb / 2 g fiber / 38 g protein

- Strip the kale from the stems and soak in a medium bowl filled with water until ready to use. This will help remove some of the bitterness of the kale.

- Mix together the paprika, garlic powder, cumin, and a pinch of salt and pepper in a small bowl. Sprinkle the spice mixture on both sides of the chicken breasts.

- Place a large skillet, preferably cast iron, over medium to high heat and add the olive oil. Cook the chicken until done, 4 to 5 minutes per side, transfer to a plate, and cover with aluminum foil.

- Reduce the heat to medium and, in the same pan, add the coconut oil. Add the mushrooms and sauté until browned. Add the sliced onions and sauté until the onions are slightly caramelized. Add salt and pepper to taste.

- While the mushrooms and onions are sautéing, drain the kale and chop it into slices.

- Add the kale to the mushroom and onion mixture and sauté until almost wilted.

- Add the sherry to deglaze the pan, reduce the heat to low, and let simmer until the kale is completely wilted, 5 to 7 minutes.

- Place the cooked kale and the mushroom and onion mixture on a large platter and top with the cooked chicken breast. Serve family style.

# TONY' MORN KALE SMOOTHIE

### SERVES: 1

*My wife and I have been enjoying this drink as a meal replacement even before we heard of Zero Belly. Once we fell in love with this eating program, I realized that I could slightly modify it to fit the Zero Belly requirements. The result? Even better!*

— TONY FRAGALE, BRENTWOOD, TN

½  **cup unsweetened almond milk**

1  **scoop vanilla plant-based protein powder**

½  **tsp ground cinnamon** (or to taste)

½  **frozen banana**

½  **cup chopped kale**

½  **tbsp natural, no-salt-added peanut butter**

   **Water to blend** (optional)

- Combine all of the ingredients in a blender and blend until smooth.

**PER SERVING:** 212 calories / 5 g fat / 23 g carb / 4 g fiber / 20 g protein

# ιERRI'S TURKEY SKILLET

SERVES: 6 COOK TIME: 20 MINUTES

*My husband loves this flavor combination on a pizza, so I figured, "Why not serve the toppings over rice?" This way you boost the protein and eliminate the gluten. This is a great make-ahead dish you can reheat as leftovers during the week. With lean ground turkey, extra-virgin olive oil, brightly colored veggies, leafy greens, and nutty brown rice—it's the most delicious way to meet your protein, fiber, and healthy fat requirements for a quick weekday meal!* —TERRI ONLEY, MD

1    **lb lean ground turkey** (at least 93% lean)

1    **tsp Italian seasoning**

3    **tbsp low-sodium tamari**

1    **tbsp extra-virgin olive oil**

2    **cloves garlic,** minced

1    **small yellow onion,** diced

½    **medium green bell pepper,** diced

1    **14½-oz can petite diced fire-roasted tomatoes,** no salt added

8    **oz baby crimini mushrooms,** sliced

3    **cups baby spinach**

1½    **cups cooked Brown Rice** (page 253)

¼    **cup chopped fresh cilantro** (optional)

- Heat a skillet over medium heat. Add the ground turkey and use a heatproof spoon or spatula to break it into pieces. Cook until browned, about 5 minutes.

- Add the Italian seasoning and 1 tablespoon tamari to the turkey and cook for 2 minutes more. Transfer the browned turkey to a plate lined with paper towels to drain any excess fat.

- Keep the skillet on the heat. Add the olive oil, garlic, onion, and bell pepper and sauté until tender, 2 to 3 minutes.

- Add the remaining 2 tablespoons of tamari to the skillet, along with the tomatoes and mushrooms. Cook until the tomato juices begin to boil, then reduce the heat to a simmer.

- Return the cooked ground turkey to pan. Add the baby spinach and heat until the spinach is wilted.

- Garnish with cilantro, if using. Serve with a side of brown rice.

**PER SERVING:** 222 calories / 8 g fat / 19 g carb / 2 g fiber / 19 g protein

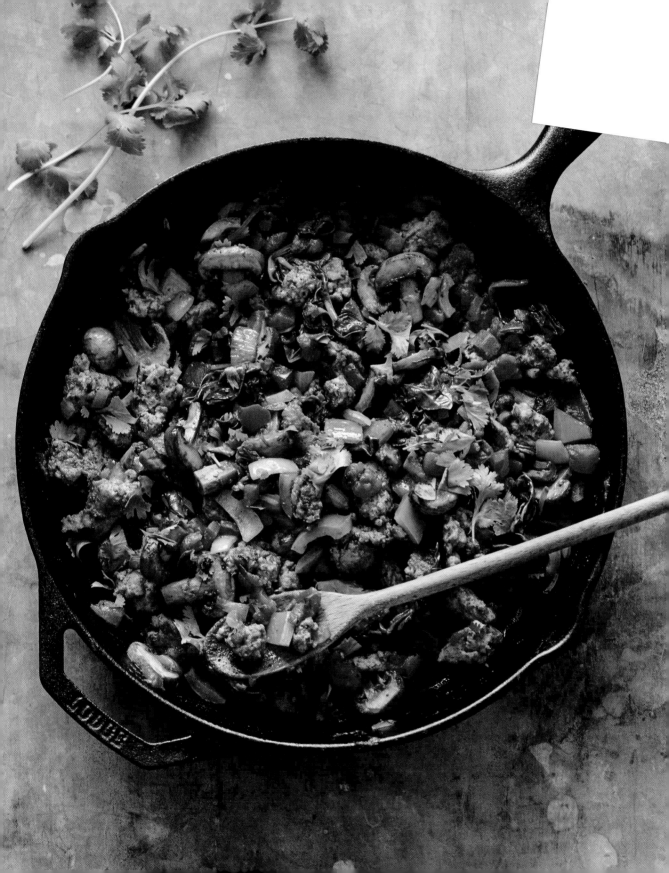

# KRISTA'S BREAKFAST SCRAMBLE

SERVES: 4   COOK TIME: 5 MINUTES

*I love this quick breakfast. It's got veggies, healthy fats, and high protein and you can adjust the heat levels with the salsa. It keeps me full until lunchtime!*

**—KRISTA POWELL, YUCAIPA, CA**

4   large eggs

4   large egg whites

 Salt and freshly ground black pepper to taste

½   tsp extra-virgin olive oil

1   red bell pepper, diced

4   oz low-sodium deli turkey, diced

1   avocado, diced

1   cup Salsa (page 245), or store-bought

- In a large bowl, whisk together the eggs, egg whites, and a pinch of salt and pepper.

- Heat the olive oil in a large nonstick pan over medium heat. Add the bell pepper and cook until softened, about 2 minutes.

- Add the turkey to the pan and cook for 30 seconds more.

- Add the whisked eggs to the pan and scramble to desired consistency.

- Divide among four bowls. Top each bowl with one-quarter of the avocado and ¼ cup salsa.

**PER SERVING:** 237 calories / 13 g fat / 12 g carb / 4 g fiber / 17 g protein

# KIM'S SAUCY SWORDFISH and SALSA

**SERVES: 4   COOK TIME: 15 MINUTES**

*I love to experiment in the kitchen, especially since reading Zero Belly Diet. The protein–fiber–healthy fat formula makes creating delicious, healthy recipes easy. This dish came about one night when I was feeling particularly creative. It's now a regularly requested dinner in my household! (Definitely don't skimp on the fruit-flavored balsamic; it makes the meal!)*

**—KIMBERLY KREAMER, PATCHOGUE, NY**

*Salsa*

- ½ **cup mango** (fresh or frozen and thawed), diced
- ½ **cup blueberries** (fresh or frozen and thawed)
- ½ **cup strawberries** (fresh or frozen and thawed), diced
- 1 **whole avocado,** diced
- ¼ **cup organic sweet corn** (fresh or frozen and thawed)
- ¼ **red onion,** diced
- ¼ **cup chopped fresh cilantro**
  **Juice of 1 lime**
- 1 **tbsp red apple balsamic vinegar** (or other fruit flavor, like raspberry)
  **Salt and freshly ground black pepper to taste**

- 1 **lb swordfish steaks** (divided into 4 portions)
- 1 **tbsp extra-virgin olive oil**
- 1 **5-oz bag arugula**

- Preheat the oven to 350°F.
- Combine the salsa ingredients in a bowl and let rest in the fridge so the flavors can mingle.
- Brush the swordfish steaks with olive oil on both sides and season lightly with salt and pepper.
- Heat an oven-proof grill pan over medium heat. Add the swordfish to the pan and sear for 2 minutes on each side.
- Place the pan in the oven and cook the swordfish for 10 minutes more.
- Divide the arugula among four plates. Top with the swordfish and one-quarter of the salsa.

**PER SERVING:** 308 calories / 18 g fat / 14 g carb / 5 g fiber / 22 g protein

# CHAPTER SIX

# ZERO BELLY DINNERS

Feast Like Royalty on a Selection of
Taste-Bud-Tantalizing Foods that Will Have You
Rushing Home for Dinner Every Night

know. You're tired. The boss has been on a rampage, the kids are on a permanent sugar high, and the commute home made *The Odyssey* look like a bike ride in the park. Cooking dinner for yourself feels like a Everest-level challenge; heck, some nights you just want someone to come and spoon the food directly into your mouth.

That's why these recipes are going to save your life.

By this stage in our journey, I probably don't have to convince you of the value of cooking at home as much as you can. But just to reinforce my point, let me drop another number on you: 33 percent. That's how much your risk of being overweight increases from eating just two meals a week out at a restaurant, according to Spanish researchers. And dinners are by far the heaviest of all restaurant meals.

To help you stay on the ZERO BELLY path, we've created a combination of meals that can be cooked primarily ahead of time; others that you can whip up in no time after a long day of work; and still others that will take advantage of a long, luxurious day of foodie indulgence. These hearty meals will have you looking forward to dinner all day long.

# SEARED SCALLOPS with ROASTED FINGERLING POTATOES and RED APPLE SLAW

**SERVES: 4    COOK TIME: 30 MINUTES**

## Potatoes

- **1** lb fingerling potatoes or about 10 pieces
- **2** sprigs rosemary
- **4** sprigs thyme
- **1** tbsp extra-virgin olive oil
- **Salt and freshly ground black pepper**

## Slaw

- **1** **large red apple,** sliced into matchsticks, skin on
- **5** **stalks celery,** sliced thinly into half-moons
- **¼** **cup coarsely chopped fresh parsley**
- **2** **tbsp walnuts,** toasted in a dry pan over medium heat until fragrant (about 2 minutes) and coarsely chopped
- **½** **tsp smoked paprika**
- **3** **tbsp Zero Belly Mayonnaise** (page 242), or store-bought
- **Juice of 1 lemon**

- **16** **large sea scallops**
- **1** tbsp extra-virgin olive oil
- **Salt and freshly ground black pepper**

**PER SERVING:** 340 calories / 10 g fat / 33 g carbs / 5 g fiber / 25 g protein

- Preheat the oven to 350°F.

- Slice the fingerling potatoes in half and place in a bowl. Add the rosemary, thyme sprigs, olive oil, and a pinch of salt and pepper. Place on a nonstick rimmed baking sheet and roast in the oven for about 30 minutes, or until soft.

- While the potatoes are cooking, prepare the slaw. Place all of the ingredients in a large bowl and mix well. Store in the fridge until ready to serve.

- When the potatoes are nearly roasted, prepare the scallops. Place the scallops on a piece of paper towel and pat dry. Wet scallops won't get any color when seared. Season with a pinch of salt and pepper.

- Heat a nonstick pan over medium to high heat. Add 1 tablespoon olive oil.

- When the oil is hot, carefully place the scallops in the pan one at a time.

- Reduce the heat to medium and cook until the scallops get a golden brown crust, 3 to 4 minutes. (No color? Turn up the heat.) Once golden, flip the scallops over and cook for 3 to 4 minutes more. The scallops should be tender to the touch and not stiff.

- Divide the red apple slaw and roasted potatoes among four plates. Discard the thyme and rosemary sprigs from the potatoes. Place three cooked scallops on top of the slaw.

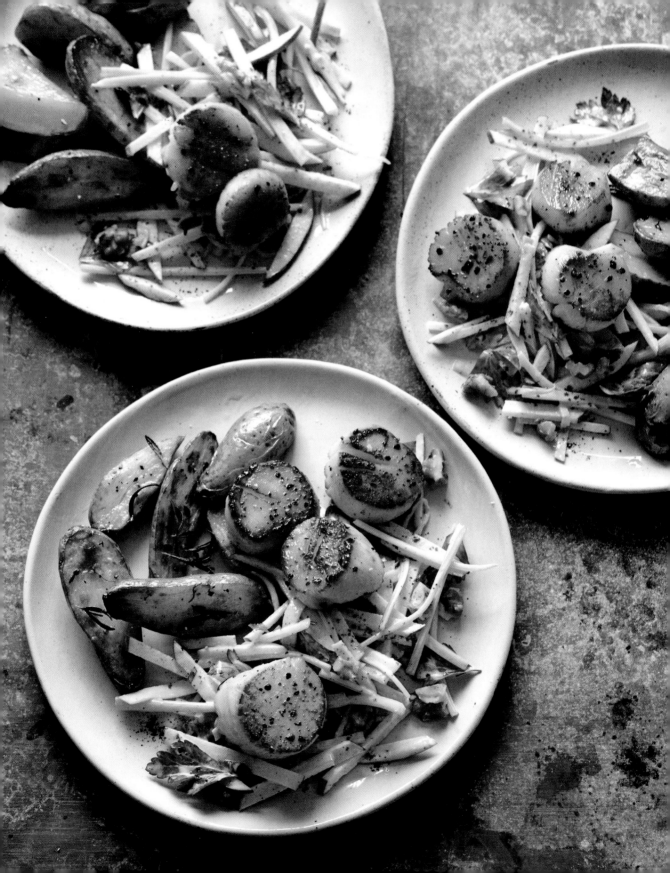

# MINI CRAB CAKE "PO BOYS" with SWEET POTATO FRIES

SERVES: 4 | COOK TIME: 40 MINUTES

## Crab Cakes
- ½ **red bell pepper,** minced
- ½ **yellow bell pepper,** minced
- 1 **red onion,** minced
- ¼ **cup gluten-free breadcrumbs**
- 3 **tbsp Zero Belly Mayonnaise** (page 242), or store-bought
- 3 **dashes Tabasco** (optional)
- 1 **tsp Dijon mustard**
- ¼ **cup almond meal**
- 1 **large egg white**
- ¼ **tsp salt**
- ¼ **tsp freshly ground black pepper**
- 1 **lb crab meat**
- 2 **tbsp extra-virgin olive oil**

## Sweet Potato Fries
- 20 **oz sweet potato**
- ½ **tbsp extra-virgin olive oil**
- ½ **tsp dried thyme**
- ½ **tsp dried rosemary**
- ½ **tsp ground cumin**

## Aioli
- ¼ **cup Zero Belly Mayonnaise** (page 242), or store-bought
- **Juice of ½ lemon**
- ¾ **tsp smoked paprika**
- ½ **tbsp relish**

## Toppings
- 1 **head Bibb lettuce**
- 1 **large tomato,** thinly sliced
- ½ **avocado,** thinly sliced

- In a large bowl, combine all of the ingredients for the crab cakes except for the crab and the oil and mix well with a rubber spatula. Then carefully fold in the crab.

- Use your hands to form 12 crab cakes. Flatten the crab cakes between the palms of your hands to about ¾-inch thickness. Set aside.

- Preheat the oven to 400°F.

- Cut each sweet potato in half lengthwise, and then into wedges. In a large bowl, combine the potatoes, olive oil, and spices. Toss evenly to coat.

- Spread the potatoes in a single layer on a rimmed baking sheet. Bake for about 35 minutes, until crisp.

- Meanwhile, heat oil in a pan over medium-high heat.

- Use a wide spatula to carefully place each crab cake in the pan. Sear for 3 minutes, or until lightly browned. Flip each cake over, and cook for 3 minutes more. Transfer the cooked crab cakes to a rimmed baking sheet. Reheat in the oven with the fries 5 minutes prior to serving.

- To prepare the aioli, mix together all of the ingredients in a small bowl.

- To assemble the "po boys": Place each crab cake on a lettuce leaf and top with dollop of aioli, a slice of tomato, and a slice of avocado.

- Divide the hot fries among four plates and serve with three "po boys."

**PER SERVING (3 crab cakes):** 480 calories / 25 g fat / 33 g carb / 6 g fiber / 29 g protein

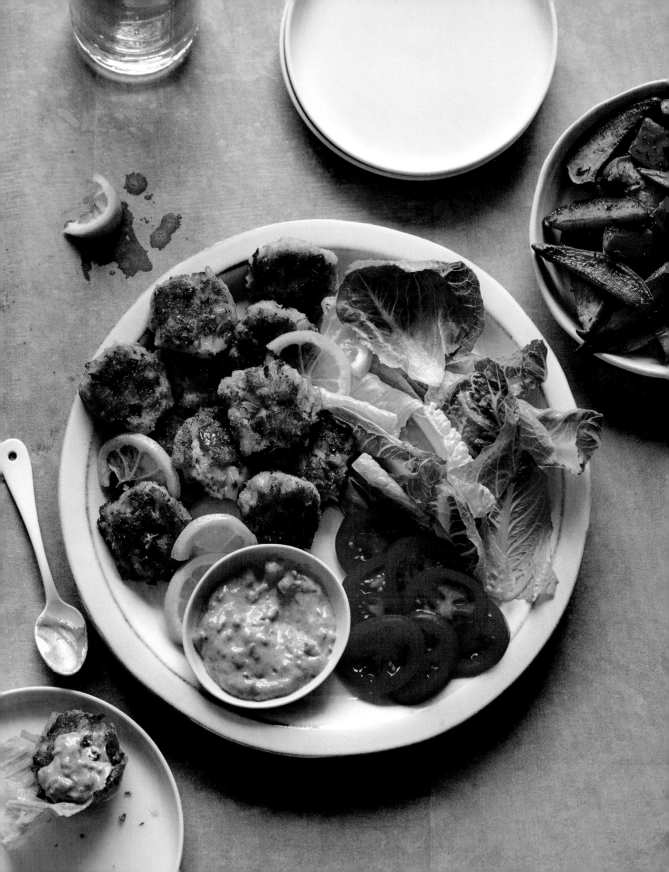

# PESTO CRUSTED SALMON with QUINOA and POMEGRANATE SALAD

SERVES: 4    COOK TIME: 20 MINUTES

4   **5-oz wild salmon fillets**

**Salt and freshly ground black pepper**

2   **tbsp Pesto**
(page 242),
or store-bought

*Salad*

1   **cup Quinoa**
(page 251)

3   **tbsp raw walnuts,**
toasted in a dry pan
over medium heat
until fragrant (about
2 minutes) and coarsely
chopped

¼   **cup dried tart cherries**

¼   **cup pomegranate seeds**

2   **tbsp Zero Belly Vinaigrette**
(page 236)

- Preheat the oven to 350°F.

- Place the salmon fillets on a nonstick rimmed baking sheet, skin-side up. Season with salt and pepper. Spread 1½ teaspoons pesto on top of each fillet.

- Place the salmon in the oven. Bake for 8 to 15 minutes, depending on the thickness of the fillets.

- Combine the salad ingredients in a large bowl. Mix well and divide among four plates.

- Top each salad with a fillet of salmon.

**PER SERVING:** 455 calories / 24 g fat / 29 g carbs / 4 g fiber / 32 g protein

# GREEN TEA–POACHED SALMON with BOK CHOY

SERVES: 4    COOK TIME: 25 MINUTES

*Poaching Liquid*

- **2  qt water**
- **5  tbsp loose green tea,** or 5 green tea bags
- **1  2-inch piece of fresh ginger,** peeled and sliced thin
- **3  tbsp low-sodium tamari**
- **Juice of 2 limes**
- **Zest of 1 orange**
- **¼  cup raw Manuka honey**
- **Salt and freshly ground black pepper to taste**

- **4  5-oz portions of wild salmon**
- **Salt and freshly ground black pepper**
- **2  tbsp extra-virgin olive oil**
- **1  lb bok choy,** cored and sliced lengthwise
- **1  tbsp water**
- **3  tbsp Zero Belly Sofrito** (page 238)
- **1  large orange**

- To prepare the poaching liquid, bring the water to a simmer in a large pot. Add the green tea, ginger, tamari, lime juice, orange zest, and honey. Do not let the poaching liquid come to a boil. Let the tea steep for 10 minutes.

- While the poaching liquid simmers, season the fish with salt and pepper and set aside.

- Once the broth has simmered for 10 minutes, turn off the heat. Season the liquid with salt and pepper to taste; it should be very flavorful.

- Place the salmon in the pot and allow to poach in the hot liquid, off the heat, for 7 to 8 minutes.

- While the salmon is poaching, heat a large sauté pan over medium heat. Add the olive oil and the bok choy to the pan. Add a tablespoon of water to the pan to help the leafy greens steam.

- Add the sofrito to the pan. Cook the bok choy until tender—4 to 5 minutes total, turning every 1 or 2 minutes.

- Divide the bok choy among four plates. Use a slotted spoon to carefully lift the salmon out of the poaching liquid. Place on top of the bok choy. Squeeze the juice of one orange on top of all four fillets. Serve immediately.

**PER SERVING:** 413 calories / 16 g fat / 34 g carb / 4 g fiber / 34 g protein

# BAKED SALMON with BEETS, CITRUS, AVOCADO, and CARAWAY SEEDS

**SERVES: 4** **COOK TIME: 10 MINUTES**

*Salmon*

4 **5-oz portions of fresh wild salmon**

**Salt and freshly ground black pepper**

*Salad*

4 **large store-bought pre-roasted beets** (not canned),* cut into bite-size pieces

3 **large oranges,** segmented

1 **Ruby Red grapefruit,** segmented

1 **cup chopped fresh parsley**

1 **tbsp caraway seeds,** toasted in a dry pan over medium heat until fragrant (about 2 minutes)

½ **avocado, diced**

2 **tbsp Zero Belly Vinaigrette** (page 236)

2 **tbsp raw walnuts,** toasted in a dry pan over medium heat until fragrant (about 2 minutes) and coarsely chopped

**Salt and freshly ground black pepper to taste**

- Preheat the oven to 350°F.

- Season the fish with a pinch of salt and pepper. Place on a nonstick rimmed baking sheet, skin-side up, and place in the oven. Cook for 6 to 8 minutes.

- Combine the salad ingredients in a large bowl. Mix well, season with salt and pepper, and divide among four plates.

- Top each salad with a 5-ounce portion of cooked salmon.

**TIP** Prefer to roast your own beets? Preheat the oven to 350°F. Wrap each large beet in a piece of foil. Place on a rimmed baking sheet and roast for about 1 hour, or until tender and easily pierced with a paring knife. Be careful not to overcook. When the beets are cool enough to handle, but still hot, use a paper towel and a paring knife to peel the beets. Plastic gloves will prevent the beet juice from staining your skin.

**PER SERVING:** 428 calories / 20 g fat / 30 g carb / 8 g fiber / 33 g protein

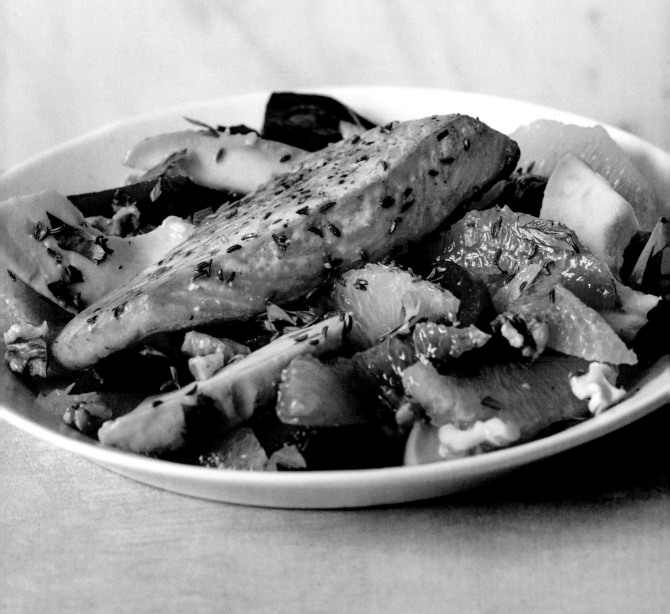

# BLACK PEPPER SHRIMP with CREAMY OATS, CHERRY TOMATOES, and ASPARAGUS

**SERVES: 4** | **COOK TIME: 40 MINUTES**

- 1 **lb large shrimp,** peeled, deveined, and heads removed (about 20 pieces)
- ¼ **cup Black Pepper Marinade** (page 239)
- 2 **cups low-sodium vegetable broth**
- 1 **tsp salt**
- 1 **cup steel cut oats**
- 1 **tbsp extra-virgin olive oil**
- 1 **bunch green asparagus,** white part of stems removed (about 20 spears)
- ¼ **cup water**
- ½ **bunch fresh cilantro,** coarsely chopped
- ½ **cup cherry tomatoes,** sliced in half
- ½ **avocado,** sliced into ¼-inch cubes

- Place the shrimp in a bowl with the marinade and mix well. Cover and allow to marinate in the fridge for at least 1 hour or overnight.

- In a medium pot, bring the vegetable broth and salt to a boil and reduce to low heat. Add the oats and cook over low heat, stirring every 2 minutes. Cook for about 30 minutes or until tender and creamy. If the oats get too thick, add more vegetable stock or water. Turn off the heat and cover with a lid to keep warm.

- Heat the olive oil in a large sauté pan over medium heat. Add the shrimp to the pan. Cook on one side for about 2 minutes. Shake the pan every 30 seconds to make sure the shrimp don't stick. Use a pair of tongs to flip the shrimp and cook for 2 minutes more, shaking the pan to prevent sticking.

- While the shrimp are cooking, bring a medium pot of water to a boil, add the asparagus, and cook for about 2 minutes or until tender. Remove the asparagus from the pot using a slotted spoon or a pair of tongs.

- Once the shrimp have cooked, add ¼ cup of water to deglaze the pan. Turn off the heat, add the cilantro, tomatoes, and avocado, and mix well.

- Divide the cooked oats among four plates. Top with the shrimp, sliced tomatoes, and avocado. Serve with a side of asparagus.

**PER SERVING:** 355 calories / 10 g fat / 35 g carb / 7 g fiber / 32 g protein

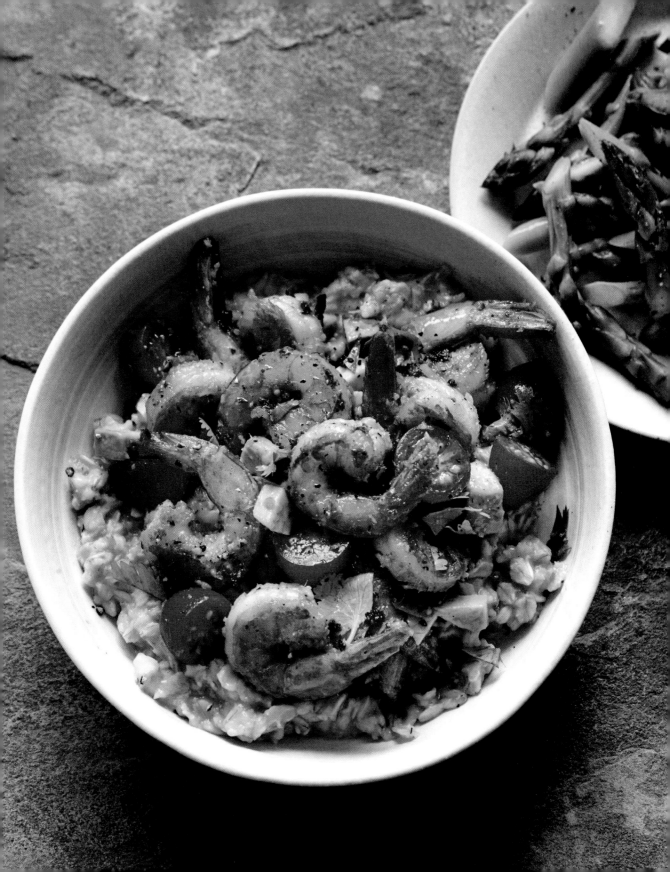

# TUNA FISH LETTUCE WRAPS with STRAWBERRY SPINACH SALAD

**SERVES: 4**  **COOK TIME: N/A**

## Tuna Wraps

1 **16-oz chunk light canned tuna,** drained

¼ **cup Zero Belly Mayonnaise** (page 242), or store-bought

½ **avocado,** diced

2 **hard-boiled eggs,** (page 250), diced

½ **medium red onion,** sliced thin

**Salt and freshly ground black pepper**

12 **Bibb lettuce leaves*** (about 1 head)

## Salad

2 **cups packed baby spinach**

1 **cup strawberries,** quartered

2 **tbsp Zero Belly Vinaigrette** (page 236)

2 **tbsp raw walnuts,** toasted in a dry pan over medium heat until fragrant (about 2 minutes) and coarsely chopped

- Place the tuna in a medium bowl and use a spatula to fold in the mayonnaise, taking care not to break up the tuna too much. Gently fold in the avocado, hard-boiled eggs, onion, and a pinch of salt and pepper to taste.

- Place a spoonful of the tuna into a Bibb lettuce leaf and place on a plate. Repeat with the remaining tuna mixture and lettuce leaves, about 12 wraps total.

- Combine all of the salad ingredients in a bowl and mix well.

- Divide the salad among four plates. Serve with three lettuce wraps.

 **TIP** Save Your Hearts! Use up leftover lettuce hearts in Seared Tuna with Lettuce Heart Salad on page 84.

**PER SERVING:** 304 calories / 15 g fat / 9 g carb / 6 g fiber / 24 g protein

# FISH and CHIPS

SERVES: 4 · COOK TIME: 35 MINUTES

### Chips

1 **lb Idaho potatoes**
(about 2 large)

1 **tbsp extra-virgin olive oil**

½ **tsp dried thyme**

½ **tsp dried rosemary**

½ **tsp ground cumin**

### Fish

1 **cup gluten-free breadcrumbs**

1 **tbsp garlic powder**
(optional)

1 **tbsp onion powder**
(optional)

4 **5-oz portions of whitefish**
(halibut or Pacific cod)

1 **large egg white,**
whisked

1 **bunch green asparagus,**
white part of
stems removed
(about 20 spears)

¼ **cup Tartar Sauce**
(page 243),
or store-bought

- Preheat the oven to 400°F.

- Peel the potatoes, cut each in half lengthwise, and cut each half into six wedges. In a large bowl, combine the potato wedges, olive oil, and spices. Toss to evenly coat the potatoes.

- Spread the chips in a single layer on a nonstick rimmed baking sheet. Bake on the middle shelf in the oven until the edges are crisp and the potatoes are cooked through, about 30 minutes.

- While the potatoes are cooking, prepare the fish. Place the breadcrumbs and garlic powder and onion powder, if desired, in a shallow bowl and toss to combine.

- Brush each fish fillet with egg white and roll in the spiced breadcrumbs, pressing firmly to ensure that the breading sticks.

- When the potatoes have about 15 minutes left of cooking time, place the fish on a nonstick rimmed baking sheet and bake for 15 minutes, or until crispy.

- While the fish and chips are cooking, bring a large pot of water to a boil. Add the asparagus and cook until tender, about 3 minutes.

- Divide the fish, chips, and asparagus among four plates and serve with 1 tablespoon tartar sauce.

**PER SERVING:** 373 calories / 12 g fat / 39 g carb / 3 g fiber / 29 g protein

# PAN-SEARED HALIBUT with CHICKPEAS, CUCUMBERS, and CHERRY TOMATOES

**SERVES: 4    COOK TIME: 10 MINUTES**

4   **5-oz portions of halibut**

**Salt and freshly ground black pepper**

1   **tbsp extra-virgin olive oil**

*Salad*

1   **cup canned chickpeas,** drained and rinsed

1   **English cucumber,** cut in half lengthwise, then sliced into half-moons

1   **cup cherry tomatoes,** halved

½   **avocado,** diced into ¼-inch cubes

1   **red pepper,** diced into ¼-inch cubes

2   **sprigs mint,** coarsely chopped

¼   **cup chopped fresh parsley**

¼   **cup Kalamata olives,** pits removed, halved

2   **tsp whole cumin seeds,** toasted in a dry pan over medium heat until fragrant (about 2 minutes)

2   **cups fresh baby spinach,** packed

2   **tbsp Zero Belly Vinaigrette** (page 236)

**Salt and freshly ground black pepper to taste**

- Season the halibut with a pinch of salt and pepper on both sides.

- Heat the olive oil in a nonstick pan over medium heat. Add halibut to the pan and cook until the fish starts to turn brown, about 3 minutes. Flip over the fish and cook for 5 minutes more, or until the fish is firm to the touch.

- Combine the salad ingredients in a large bowl. Mix well, season with salt and pepper, and divide among four plates.

- Top each salad with a 5-ounce portion of halibut.

**PER SERVING:** 375 calories / 17 g fat / 21 g carb / 6 g fiber / 35 g protein

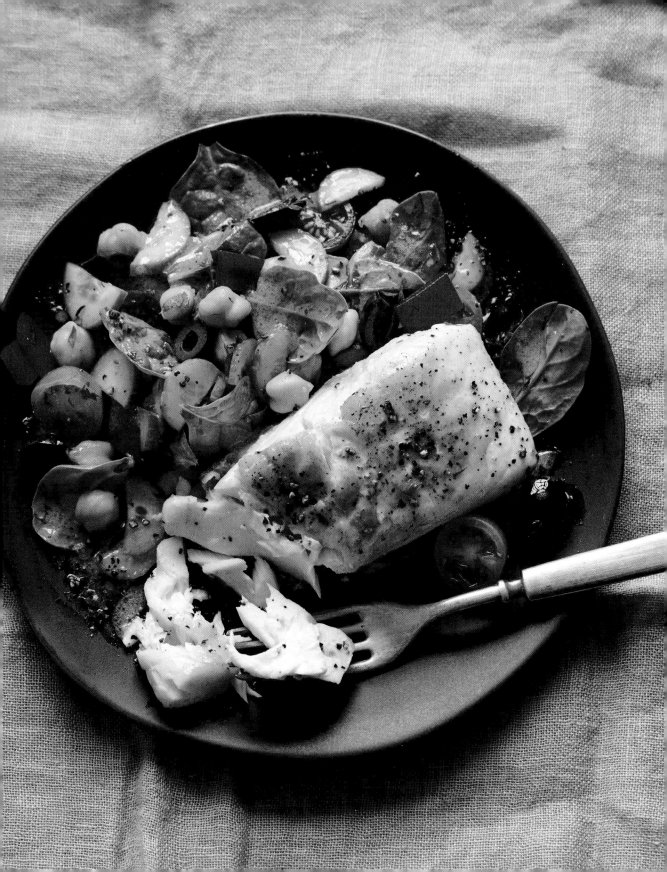

# SPICE-CRUSTED TUNA with TOMATO and BEAN RAGOUT

SERVES: 4    COOK TIME: 20 MINUTES

*Ragout*

2   tbsp extra-virgin olive oil

1   small yellow onion, coarsely chopped

1   large red bell pepper, coarsely chopped

4   cloves garlic, minced

½   cup canned pinto beans, drained and rinsed

½   cup canned kidney beans, drained and rinsed

½   cup canned garbanzo beans, drained and rinsed

8   oz no-salt-added diced tomatoes

½   tbsp freshly ground black pepper

2   tsp kosher salt

3   tbsp coarsely chopped fresh parsley

2   tbsp coarsely chopped fresh oregano (optional)

3   tbsp coarsely chopped fresh chives (optional)

1   lb Seared Tuna (page 248)

- Cook the ragout. Place the olive oil, onions, bell pepper, and garlic in a saucepan and cook over medium heat until softened, about 5 minutes. Add the beans and the tomatoes with the juice. Bring to a boil, reduce the heat to a simmer, and cook, covered, for 10 minutes more. Add the pepper, salt, and herbs. Mix well.

- Sear the tuna (page 248).

- Divide the ragout among four bowls and top with 4 ounces seared, sliced tuna.

**PER SERVING:** 287 calories / 9 g fat / 18 g carb / 5 g fiber / 32 g protein

# TURKEY BURGERS with PESTO and ROASTED RED PEPPERS

SERVES: 4    COOK TIME: 20 MINUTES

1   lb extra-lean ground turkey (99%)

2   tbsp whole-grain mustard

1   tsp salt

½   tsp freshly ground black pepper

4   gluten-free burger buns

2   tbsp Pesto (page 242)

4   pieces jarred roasted red peppers, thinly sliced

8   Bibb or Boston lettuce leaves, rinsed and blotted dry

- In a large bowl, mix together the ground turkey, mustard, salt, and pepper. Let sit for 10 minutes.

- While the turkey is marinating, heat an outdoor grill or grill pan over medium-high heat.

- Form the turkey mixture into 4 patties and grill for 3 to 4 minutes on each side. The center should be fully cooked but still juicy.

- Toast the burger buns until golden brown.

- Spread each toasted burger bun top with 1½ teaspoons pesto.

- Place a burger on each toasted burger bun bottom, and top with one sliced red pepper, two lettuce leaves, and a pesto-spread burger bun top.

**PER SERVING:** 370 calories / 13 g fat / 38 g carb / 2 g fiber / 26 g protein

# CHICKEN PROVENÇAL with SWISS CHARD and BROWN RICE

SERVES: 4    COOK TIME: 25 MINUTES

Olive oil spray

4   5-oz skinless, boneless chicken breasts

Salt and freshly ground black pepper

2   cups Marinara (page 241), or store-bought

½   lb Swiss chard,* rinsed of dirt and patted dry

1   tbsp extra-virgin olive oil

¼   cup water

½   lemon

2   cups Brown Rice (page 253)

½   cup coarsely chopped fresh basil (optional)

Mustard greens or bok choy can be used as a replacement.

- Preheat the oven to 350°F.

- Heat a nonstick pan, lightly coated with olive oil spray, over medium heat.

- Season the chicken breast with a pinch of salt and pepper, and sear in the pan until lightly golden brown, about 3 minutes on each side. Don't worry about cooking the chicken breast all the way through. Place the seared chicken in a glass casserole dish.

- Pour the marinara over the chicken breasts and cover the dish with aluminum foil. Place in the oven and cook for 15 minutes.

- While the chicken cooks, prepare the Swiss chard. Coarsely chop the green leaves of the stems. Thinly slice the stems and set aside.

- Heat the olive oil in a large sauté pan over medium heat. Add the Swiss chard stems and sauté until tender, about 2 minutes. Add the Swiss chard leaves and add the water. Steam until tender, about 2 minutes. Finish with a squeeze of half a lemon.

- Divide the cooked Swiss chard among four plates. Top with one chicken breast and marinara. Serve with ½ cup brown rice. Garnish with basil, if desired.

**PER SERVING:** 300 calories / 3 g fat / 38 g carbs / 6 g fiber / 39 g protein

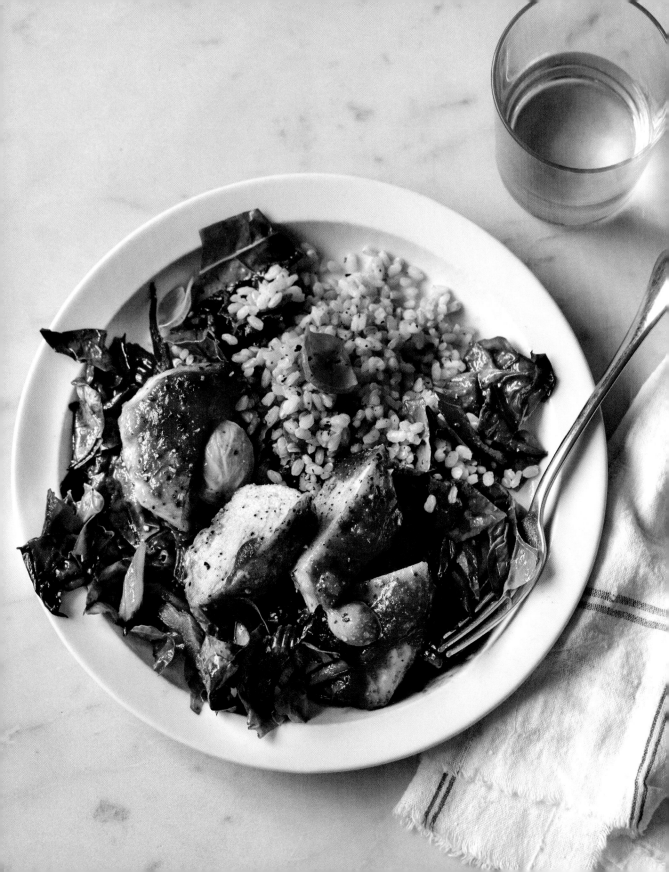

# MARINATED LAMB CHOPS with WHOLE-GRAIN-MUSTARD POTATOES and KALE

**SERVES: 4** | **COOK TIME: 40 MINUTES**

## Marinade

- ¼ cup **extra-virgin olive oil**
- 2 **cloves garlic,** peeled and smashed
- 1½ tsp **fresh rosemary leaves**
- 1½ tsp **fresh thyme leaves**
- 3 **sprigs fresh mint**
- 1 tbsp **whole coriander seed** (optional)
- 2 tbsp **(packed) brown sugar**
- 1 tsp **freshly ground black pepper**

- 8 **4-oz lamb loin chops,** trimmed of all visible fat
  **Salt**
- 2 tbsp **extra-virgin olive oil**

**Whole-Grain-Mustard Potato Salad** (page 144)

**Wilted Kale Salad** (page 140)

- Place all of the marinade ingredients in the bowl of a food processor, then pulse until lightly chopped (do not puree).

- Place the chops in a large bowl and pour the marinade over them. Move the chops around in the bowl so that the marinade coats them well. Cover the bowl with plastic wrap and marinate for at least 4 hours; 12 hours would be ideal.

- Preheat the oven to 400°F.

- Scrape the marinade off the lamb, place the lamb on a plate or a rimmed baking sheet, season lightly with salt, and let sit at room temperature for 20 minutes.

- Meanwhile, prepare the Whole-Grain-Mustard Potato Salad and Wilted Kale Salad.

- Once the lamb has reached room temperature, heat a large sauté pan or grill pan over medium-high heat. Add 2 tablespoons olive oil to the pan. Grill or broil the chops for 3 to 4 minutes per side for medium rare.

- Divide the potatoes and kale among four plates and serve with two lamb chops.

**PER SERVING:** 462 calories / 20 g fat / 27 g carb / 3 g fiber / 2 g protein

# GRILLED STEAK with CHILLED ASPARAGUS SALAD

SERVES: 4 COOK TIME: 5 MINUTES

1 **bunch green asparagus,** white part of stems removed (about 20 spears)

1 **lb Grilled Steak** (page 249)

*Sauce Gribiche*

6 **cornichons,** quartered

1 **egg,** hard-boiled (page 250)

1 **tsp Dijon mustard**

1 **tbsp red wine vinegar**

¼ **cup extra-virgin olive oil**

¼ **cup chopped mixed fresh herbs** (parsley, chive, tarragon)

**Salt and freshly ground black pepper**

¼ **cup baby arugula** (optional)

- Blanch the asparagus. Bring a large pot of water to a boil. Meanwhile, fill a large bowl with ice and cold water. Drop the asparagus in the boiling water and cook for 1 to 2 minutes. Use a slotted spoon to transfer the spears from the hot water directly into the ice bath to cool. Drain the blanched asparagus in a colander and transfer to a plate covered with paper towel to dry completely.

- Grill the steak and set aside to rest.

- Prepare the Sauce Gribiche. In the bowl of a food processor, add the cornichons and the egg. Pulse a few times until coarsely chopped. Do not overpulse.

- In a separate bowl, whisk together the mustard, vinegar, and olive oil. Whisk in the chopped eggs, cornichons, and the mixed herbs.

- Slice and divide the grilled steak among four plates. Arrange the chilled asparagus alongside the steak, tips facing the same direction. Spoon the Sauce Gribiche on the asparagus, season with a pinch of salt and pepper, and garnish with fresh arugula, if using.

**PER SERVING:** 373 calories / 29 g fat / 3 g carb / 2 g fiber / 25 g protein

# TURKEY MEATLOAF MUFFINS with APPLE CIDER–DIJON GLAZE and WILTED KALE SALAD

**SERVES: 4     COOK TIME: 30 MINUTES**

- 1  **lb ground turkey breast** (93% or leaner)
- ¼  **cup old-fashioned rolled oats**
- ½  **cup finely chopped onions**
- 2  **cloves garlic,** minced
- 1  **tbsp Zero Belly Sofrito** (page 238)
- 2  **tbsp low-sodium Worcestershire sauce**
- 2  **tbsp ketchup**
- 1  **large egg white**

*Glaze*
- ¼  **cup apple cider**
- 3  **tbsp raw Manuka honey**
- 4  **tsp Dijon mustard**

*Salad*
- 1  **bunch of Tuscan kale,** rinsed, dried, and coarsely chopped
- 1  **tbsp Zero Belly Vinaigrette** (page 236)
- ¼  **cup grape tomatoes**
- 2  **tbsp raw walnuts,** toasted in a dry pan over medium heat until fragrant (about 2 minutes)

- Preheat the oven to 350°F.
- In the bowl of a food processor or large bowl, add the turkey, oats, onions, garlic, sofrito, Worcestershire, ketchup, and egg white. Pulse or mix until just combined. Do not overmix.
- Roll the mixture into 8 individual balls and place them into 8 holes of a standard 12-hole muffin tin.
- For the glaze, whisk together the apple cider, honey, and mustard in a small bowl. Pour half the glaze into a fresh bowl and set aside.
- Brush the top of the uncooked turkey muffins with half of the glaze and place in the oven.
- Cook for 15 minutes. Remove the pan from the oven and use a clean brush and the remaining glaze to brush the cooked muffins. Cook for 15 minutes more.
- When the muffins have about 10 minutes left of cooking time, toss the kale and vinaigrette and set aside.
- Transfer the muffin pan to a cooling rack and let sit for at least 5 minutes. Right before serving, mix the grape tomatoes and the walnuts into the salad.
- Divide the salad among four plates along with two meatloaf muffins.

**PER SERVING:**
349 calories / 13 g fat / 31 g carb / 3 g fiber / 30 g protein (with 93% lean ground turkey)

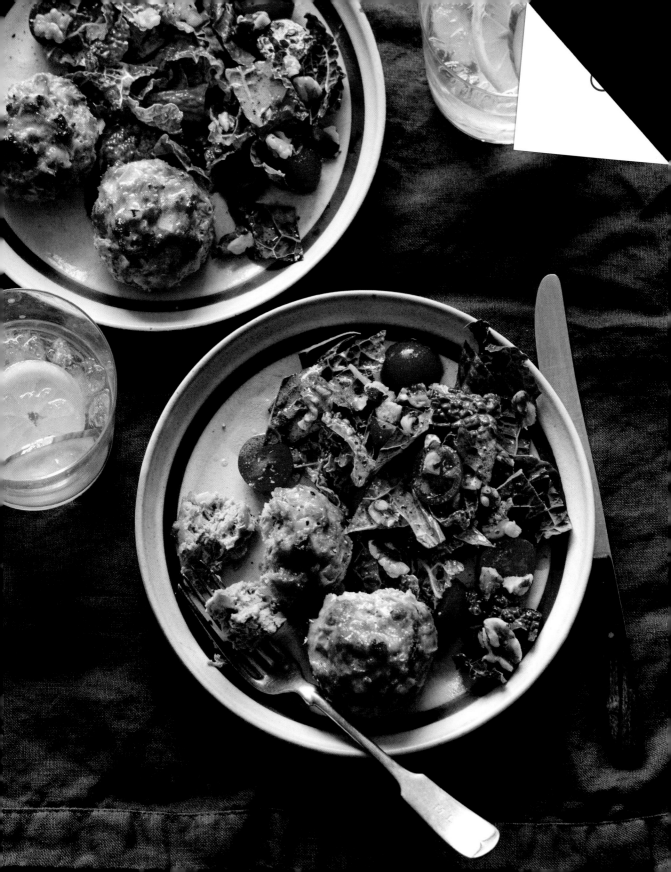

# GRILLED CHICKEN FAJITAS with BIBB LETTUCE WRAPS

**SERVES: 4** | **COOK TIME: 30 MINUTES**

- **20** oz skinless, boneless chicken breasts
- **2** tbsp Mexican Spice Blend (page 240)
- **1** large white onion, cut into ½-inch-thick rings
- **2** large red bell peppers, cut into ½-inch-thick strips
- **2** heads Bibb lettuce leaves
- **½** cup Salsa (page 245), or store-bought
- **1** cup Guacamole (page 243)

- Heat a grill or grill pan over high heat.

- Rub the chicken with the spice blend. Let sit for 5 minutes.

- Place the chicken breasts on the grill using a pair of tongs and let sit until marked, 3 to 4 minutes. Quarter-turn the chicken on the same side and repeat. Turn the chicken breasts over and let sit on the grill, undisturbed, for 3 to 4 minutes.

- Meanwhile, place the onion rings and bell peppers on the grill.

- Quarter-turn the chicken on the same side and let cook for 3 to 4 minutes more. Pull the chicken off the grill and let rest.

- Turn the onions and peppers a few times, until tender.

- Cut the grilled chicken breasts into strips. Place the grilled chicken and vegetable strips on a platter and serve, family style, with Bibb lettuce leaf "wraps," salsa, and guacamole.

**PER SERVING:** 257 calories / 10 g fat / 17 g carbs / 6 g fiber / 29 g protein

# MULLIGATAWNY SOUP

SERVES: 4    COOK TIME: 45 MINUTES

- **1 tbsp extra-virgin olive oil**
- **1 lb skinless, boneless chicken breasts,** cut into 1-inch cubes
- **1 large yellow onion,** finely diced
- **1 large carrot,** finely diced
- **1 red bell pepper,** finely diced
- **6 cloves garlic,** sliced thin
- **1 cup celery root,** finely diced
- **2 tbsp Zero Belly Sofrito** (page 238)
- **1 tbsp curry powder**
- **1 tsp paprika**
- **1 qt low-sodium chicken broth**
- **1 14-oz can light coconut milk**
- **1 Yukon Gold potato,** peeled and finely diced
- **1 cinnamon stick**
- **2 tbsp natural, no-salt-added peanut butter**
- **½ bunch fresh mint and ½ bunch fresh thyme,** tied together with a string
- **1 dried bay leaf**
- **1 lime**

- Heat the olive oil in large saucepan over medium heat. Add the chicken and brown all sides using a pair of tongs, about 4 to 5 minutes. Once browned, transfer the chicken to a plate lined with paper towels.

- In the same pot, add the onion, carrot, bell pepper, garlic, and celery root. Cook over medium heat for 3 to 4 minutes, stirring every minute or so, so that the vegetables don't burn. Stir in the sofrito, curry powder, and paprika. Add the chicken stock and coconut milk. Bring to a simmer. Add the cooked chicken, potato, cinnamon stick, peanut butter, tied herbs, and bay leaf and stir to combine.

- Cook over low heat until the potatoes are fork tender, 15 to 20 minutes. Discard the tied herbs, bay leaf, and cinnamon stick.

- Divide among four large bowls. Finish with a squeeze of fresh lime juice.

**PER SERVING:** 370 calories / 15 g fat / 27 g carb / 5 g fiber / 31 g protein

# GRILLED CHICKEN KABOBS with WHOLE-GRAIN-MUSTARD POTATO SALAD

SERVES: 4    COOK TIME: 40 MINUTES

## Potato Salad

- 1 **lb fingerling potatoes** (about 10 potatoes), cut in half
- 2 **tbsp whole-grain mustard**
- 2 **tbsp Zero Belly Vinaigrette** (page 236)
- 2 **tbsp Zero Belly Mayonnaise** (page 242), or store-bought
- 1 **cup packed baby arugula**
- ½ **tsp salt**

## Kabobs

- 1 **lb skinless, boneless chicken breasts,** cut into 1½-inch cubes
  **Salt and freshly ground black pepper**
- 1 **red bell pepper,** cut into 1½-inch pieces
- 1 **red onion,** cut into 1½-inch pieces
- 8 **oz button mushrooms** (about 12 medium), kept whole

## Special Equipment

- 8 **bamboo skewers,** soaked in water for 10 minutes to prevent burning

**For the potato salad:**

- Place the potatoes in a saucepan and cover with cold water. Bring to a boil over high heat, then reduce the heat to medium and cook until tender, about 10 minutes.

- Strain the potatoes in a colander and place in a medium bowl. Place in the fridge to cool.

- Once cool, add the remaining potato salad ingredients to the bowl and mix to combine.

**For the kabobs:**

- Heat an outdoor grill or a grill pan over high heat.

- Season the chicken cubes lightly with a pinch of salt and pepper. Skewer the chicken cubes and sliced vegetables alternately on large skewers and place on the grill.

- Cook on all four sides until the chicken and vegetables get nice grill marks, 3 to 4 minutes per side.

- Divide the potato salad among four plates and serve with two hot chicken kabobs.

**PER SERVING:** 364 calories / 16 g fat / 26 g carb / 4 g fiber / 31 g protein

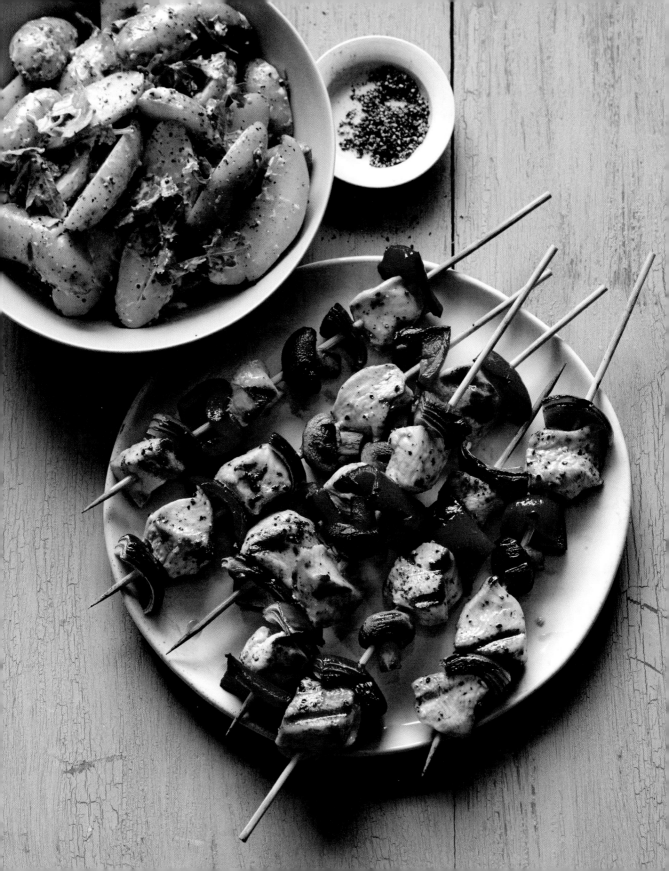

# SPAGHETTI SQUASH and MEATBALLS

**SERVES: 4**   **COOK TIME: 1 HOUR**

2  **lb spaghetti squash**
   (2 small or 1 large)

2  **cups Marinara**
   (page 241),
   or store-bought

16  **Turkey Meatballs**
   (page 247)

¼  **cup coarsely chopped fresh basil**

¼  **cup coarsely chopped fresh parsley**

- Preheat the oven to 350°F.

- Cut the spaghetti squash in half and scoop out the seeds with a spoon. Place in an oven-safe baking dish, flesh-side up, and pour about 2 tablespoons of water in each cavity. Cover with aluminum foil and bake for 50 minutes to 1 hour, until fork tender but not mushy. Remove from the oven and let rest until cool enough to handle.

- Meanwhile, add the marinara and meatballs to a saucepan over medium heat, and heat until warm, about 5 minutes. Stir every minute or so to ensure that the sauce does not burn.

- Once the squash has cooled, pour out the water and use a fork to scrape long, spaghetti-like strands from the flesh into a bowl.

- Divide the squash among four plates and top each serving with 4 meatballs and ½ cup marinara.

- Garnish with the basil and parsley.

**PER SERVING:** 300 calories / 14 g fat / 22 g carb / 2 g fiber / 20 g protein

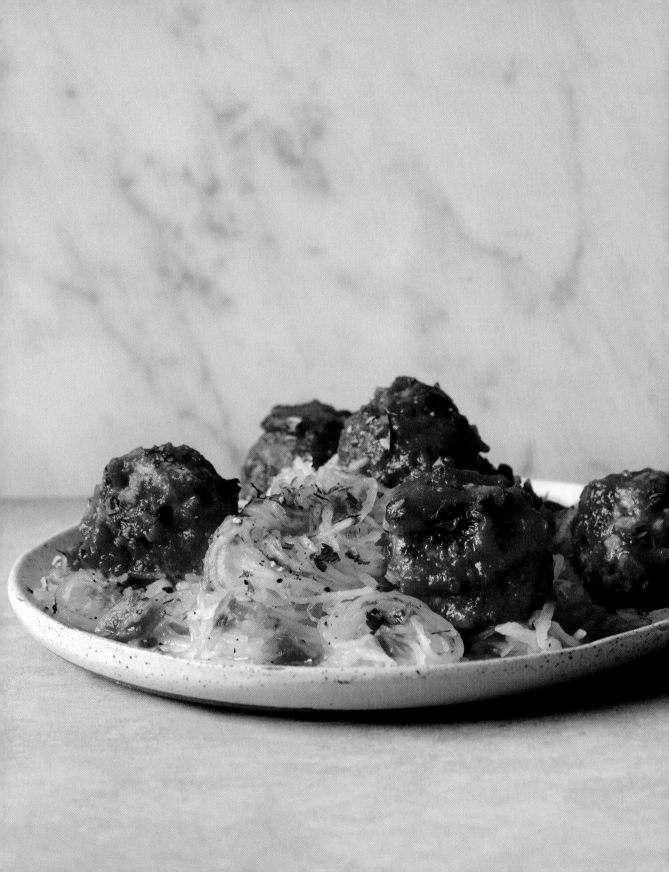

# GRILLED SIRLOIN with ONIONS, PEPPERS, and GUACAMOLE

SERVES: 4   COOK TIME: 30 MINUTES

1   **20-oz sirloin steak**

¼   **cup Black Pepper Marinade** (page 239)

   **Salt**

1   **large white onion**

2   **red bell peppers**

½   **cup Guacamole** (page 243)

1   **bunch scallions,** coarsely chopped (optional)

- Heat a grill or grill pan over high heat.

- Rub the steak with the marinade* and season lightly with a pinch of salt. Let sit for 10 minutes.

- While the steak is marinating, peel the onion and slice into rings about ⅓ inch thick. Cut the peppers into quarters and remove the seeds and the white veins.

- Place the steak on the grill using a pair of tongs and let sit until marked, 3 to 4 minutes. Quarter-turn the steak on the same side and repeat. Turn the steak over and let it sit on the grill, undisturbed, for 3 to 4 minutes.

- Meanwhile, place the onion and peppers on the grill.

- Quarter-turn the steak on the same side and let cook for 3 to 4 minutes more. Pull the steak off the grill and let rest.

- Turn over the onion and peppers a few times until tender.

- Slice the steak into strips. Divide the steak among four plates and top with the onions, peppers, and 2 tablespoons guacamole, if desired. Garnish with scallions, if using.

Short on time? Swap the Black Pepper Marinade for 1 tablespoon Mexican Spice Blend (page 240).

**PER SERVING:** 470 calories / 26 g fat / 16 g carbs / 3 g fiber / 39 g protein

# SLOW-COOKED BEEF STEW

**SERVES: 4 COOK TIME: 8 HOURS 15 MINUTES**

- 2 **tbsp extra-virgin olive oil**
- 1 **lb beef top round,** cut into 1-inch cubes
- 1 **tsp smoked paprika**
- 1 **8-oz can no-salt-added crushed tomatoes**
- 1 **qt low-sodium beef broth**
- ½ **lb fingerling potatoes,** cut in half
- 1 **12-oz can button mushrooms,** cut in half
- ½ **pound carrots** (about 2 large), split down the middle and cut into half-moons about ¼ inch thick
- 1 **small white onion,** finely diced
- 4 **cloves garlic,** sliced thin
- 1 **red bell pepper,** finely diced
- 2 **stalks celery,** sliced into half-moons, about ¼ inch thick
- ¼ **cup long-grain brown rice,** uncooked
- 1 **tsp dried thyme leaves**
- 1 **tsp dried rosemary**
- 1 **tsp kosher salt**
- 1 **tsp cracked black pepper**

- Heat a large skillet or saucepan over medium heat. Add the olive oil and cubed beef and cook undisturbed for about 3 minutes, or until the beef starts to brown slightly.

- Continue to cook, turning the beef as needed with a pair of tongs, until mostly browned on all sides, 3 to 4 minutes.

- Once browned, add the paprika and stir into the meat. Add the tomatoes (with juice) and cook for 2 minutes, or until the tomatoes have reduced by half. Transfer the beef and tomatoes to a 4-quart slow cooker along with the beef broth.*

- Add all of the remaining ingredients to the slow cooker and stir well.

- Cook for 8 hours on low to medium temperature or until the beef is very tender.

- Divide the stew among four bowls. Serve hot.

Alternatively, this stew can be cooked in a Dutch oven, lid on, for 3 hours at 250°F.

**PER SERVING:** 415 calories / 10 g fat / 26 g carb / 5 g fiber / 44 g protein

# STEAK FRITES with ARUGULA CHIMICHURRI and ASPARAGUS

SERVES: 4    COOK TIME: 35 MINUTES

## Frites

- 1   **lb russet or Idaho potatoes** (about 2 large)
- 1   **tbsp extra-virgin olive oil**
- ½   **tsp dried thyme**
- ½   **tsp dried rosemary**

## Steak

- ¼   **cup Black Pepper Marinade** (page 239)*
- 1   **20-oz flank steak,** cut into four 5-oz portions
- ½   **cup Arugula Chimichurri** (page 240)

<br>

- 1   **bunch green asparagus,** white part of stems removed (about 20 spears)

TIP   Short on time? Swap the Black Pepper Marinade for 1 tablespoon Mexican Spice Blend (page 240).

**PER SERVING:** 475 calories / 23 g fat / 32 g carb / 5 g fiber / 34 g protein

- Preheat the oven to 400°F.

- Peel the potatoes, cut each in half length-wise, and cut each half into 6 wedges. In a large bowl, combine the potato wedges, olive oil, and herbs. Toss to evenly coat the potatoes.

- Spread the frites in a single layer on a non-stick rimmed baking sheet. Bake on the middle shelf in the oven until the edges are crisp and the potatoes are cooked through, about 30 minutes.

- While the potatoes are cooking, spoon the marinade on either side of the steaks and set aside to marinate for at least 10 minutes.

- When the potatoes have about 20 minutes left of cooking time, heat a grill pan or grill over medium-high heat. Place the steaks on the hot grill using a pair of tongs and let sit, undisturbed, until the steaks get nice grill marks—3 to 4 minutes. (If you like your steak well done, let grill 5 minutes before turning.) Quarter-turn the steaks on the same side and repeat.

- Flip the steaks over and cook for 3 to 4 minutes more. Quarter-turn the steaks on the same side and repeat.

- While your steaks finish cooking, add the asparagus to the grill pan.

- Pull the steaks off the grill and let rest on a plate. Flip the asparagus over a few times until tender.

- Divide the asparagus and frites among four plates. Serve with one steak topped with 2 tablespoons chimichurri.

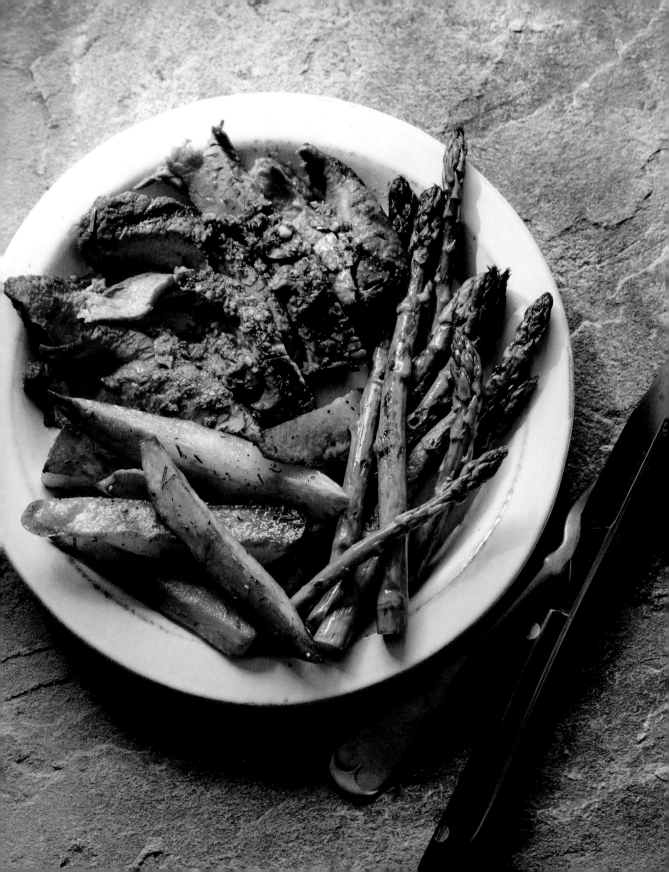

# TACO SALAD

SERVES: 4    COOK TIME: 10 MINUTES

Olive oil spray

1   lb extra-lean ground beef
    (at least 90%)

2   tbsp Mexican Spice Blend
    (page 240)

1   head iceberg lettuce,
    chopped into 1-inch cubes

1   cup Salsa
    (page 245)

½   cup Guacamole
    (page 243)

- Heat a large skillet sprayed with olive oil over medium-high heat and add the ground beef. Use a rubber spatula or a wooden spoon to break up the ground beef into small pieces until browned.

- Add the spice blend to the pan and mix well. Remove from the heat and use a slotted spoon to transfer the beef to a plate covered in paper towels to drain any excess fat.

- Divide the lettuce among four plates and top each salad with a quarter of the spicy beef. Top with ¼ cup salsa and 2 tablespoons guacamole.

**PER SERVING:** 312 calories / 17 g fat / 14 g carb / 5 g fiber / 25 g protein

# TURKEY TUSCAN VEGETABLE SOUP

SERVES: 4    COOK TIME: 30 MINUTES

2 qt low-sodium vegetable or chicken broth

½ cup finely diced onions

½ cup finely diced carrots

½ cup finely diced celery

¼ cup finely diced red bell pepper

¼ cup finely diced fennel

2 tbsp Zero Belly Sofrito (page 238)

6 sprigs fresh thyme

1 sprig fresh rosemary

2 dried bay leaves

16 Turkey Meatballs (page 247)

¾ cup canned garbanzo beans, drained and rinsed

¾ cup canned kidney beans, drained and rinsed

Salt and freshly ground black pepper

3 tbsp chopped fresh parsley

- In a large pot add the broth, vegetables, and sofrito. Bring to a boil.

- Tie the thyme, rosemary, and bay leaves together with string and add to the pot with the broth and vegetables.

- Reduce the heat to a low simmer, add the cooked meatballs, and simmer for 15 minutes.

- Remove and discard the herbs. Add the beans and season with salt and pepper to taste. Garnish with chopped parsley. Serve hot.

**PER SERVING:** 200 calories / 4 g fat / 24 g carb / 8 g fiber / 21 g protein

# CLASSIC BEEF BURGERS

**SERVES: 4   COOK TIME: 20 MINUTES**

1   **lb extra-lean ground beef** (at least 90%)

3   **tbsp Black Pepper Marinade** (page 239)

1   **tsp kosher salt**

4   **gluten-free English muffins or burger buns,** toasted

1   **beefsteak tomato,** cut into ½-inch slices

8   **leaves Bibb lettuce**

2   **tbsp ketchup**

2   **tbsp Dijon mustard**

- In a large bowl, mix the ground beef, marinade, and salt and let sit for 10 minutes.

- While the beef is marinating, heat an outdoor grill or a grill pan over medium-high heat.

- Form the beef mixture into 4 patties and grill for 2 to 3 minutes on each side. The center should be pink and juicy.

- Spread each toasted burger bun top with 1½ teaspoons ketchup and 1½ teaspoons mustard. Place a burger on each toasted burger bun bottom and top with slices of red tomato, 2 lettuce leaves, and a burger top.

**PER SERVING:** 343 calories / 9 g fat / 41 g carb / 2 g fiber / 25 g protein

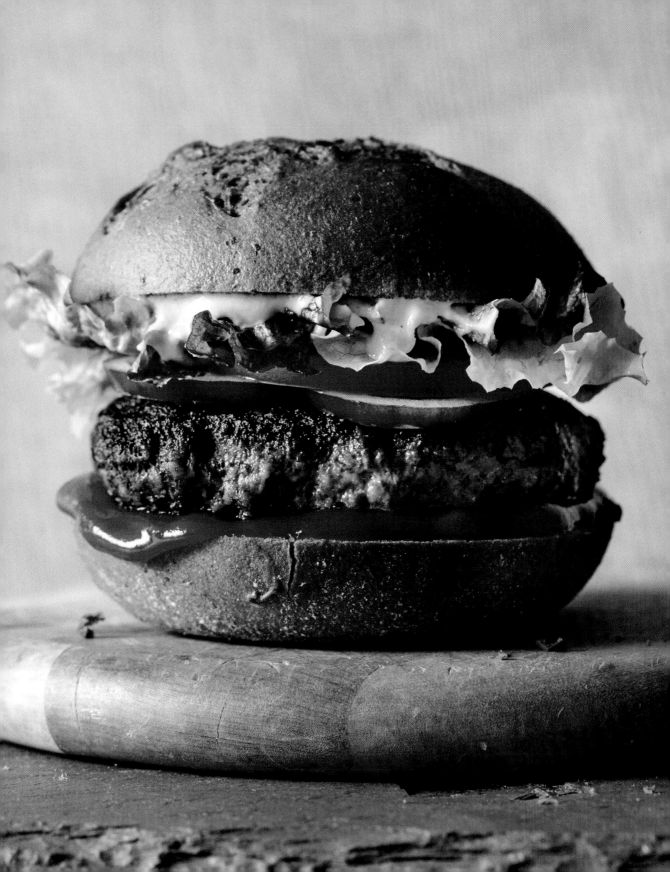

# PERFECT ROAST CHICKEN
# with ROASTED VEGETABLES

SERVES: 4    COOK TIME: 1 HOUR

## Brine

½   cup kosher salt

½   cup sugar

**Zest and juice of 1 lemon,** peeled with a vegetable peeler

**Zest and juice of 1 orange,** peeled with a vegetable peeler

2   **dried bay leaves** (optional)

8   **sprigs fresh thyme** (optional)

1   **sprig fresh rosemary** (optional)

1   **head of garlic,** cut in half

1   **tbsp freshly ground black pepper**

1   **gallon hot water**

1   **3-lb organic chicken,** giblets removed*

## Vegetables

2   **large carrots,** peeled and cut into 1-inch pieces

1   **fennel bulb,** cut in half and then into thirds

1   **large onion,** cut into 1-inch pieces

½   **lb fingerling potatoes,** cut in half

**Olive oil spray**

**Quinoa "Stuffing" with Dried Cherries and Walnuts** (optional) (page 252)

- Place all of the brine ingredients, except for the water, in a container large enough to hold the brine and the chicken. Add the gallon of hot water to the bowl and mix with a large spoon to dissolve the salt and sugar.

- Let cool to room temperature and place the chicken in the brine. Let brine overnight, for at least 8 hours and no longer than 12 hours.

- Remove the chicken from the brine and pat dry with paper towels.

- Preheat the oven to 425°F.

- Place the chicken in a roasting pan. Tie the legs together with kitchen string and tuck the wing tips under the body of the chicken. Place the cut vegetables around the chicken. Spray the chicken with olive oil spray.

- Place the roasting pan in the oven and let cook for 15 minutes. Then reduce the heat to 350°F and cook for 45 minutes more. If the chicken starts to get too much color, cover with aluminum foil.

- Check to make sure the chicken is done by cutting a slice between the leg and the breast. If the juices are clear, it's cooked. If there is still blood in the juice, cook for 10 to 15 minutes more and retest.

- Once cooked, place the chicken on a cooling rack and let it rest for 5 to 10 minutes. Divide the vegetables and stuffing, if using, among four plates. Carve the chicken and serve 5 to 6 ounces of white and dark meat per plate.

This recipe can be easily adjusted for turkey:

**8- to 10-lb turkey (serves 6 to 8):** Double the marinade, double the vegetables and stuffing, and bake for 2 hours.

**10- to 14-lb turkey (serves 8 to 10):** Double the marinade, double or triple the vegetables and stuffing, and bake for 2½ hours.

**PER SERVING:** 327 calories / 4 g fat / 21 g carb / 4 g fiber / 28 g protein

# VEGETABLE LASAGNA with BASIL PECAN PESTO

**SERVES: 4 COOK TIME: 45 MINUTES**

1 **lb eggplant** (1 to 2), sliced into rounds of ⅛-inch "noodles"

**Salt**

**Olive oil spray**

1 **lb yellow squash** (1 to 2), sliced lengthwise into ⅛-inch "noodles"

1 **lb zucchini** (1 to 2), sliced lengthwise into ⅛-inch "noodles"

1½ **cups part-skim ricotta cheese**

1 **large egg white**

⅓ **cup Pesto** (page 242), or store-bought

1 **8-oz jar roasted red pepper,** drained and sliced into strips

1½ **cups Marinara** (page 241), or store-bought

- Preheat the oven to 375°F.

- Lay the eggplant in a single layer on a rimmed baking sheet and salt generously. Allow the eggplant to sit for 30 minutes to 1 hour. Rinse with water and dry well. Spray the baking sheet with olive oil spray; spread eggplant out in a single layer and spray with more olive oil. Place in the oven for 5 minutes.

- While the eggplant cooks, spray another rimmed baking sheet with olive oil. Spread a single layer of yellow squash and zucchini slices. After the eggplant has cooked for 5 minutes, add the baking sheet with yellow squash and zucchini to the oven. Bake for 5 minutes more. Remove both trays from the oven.

- While the vegetables are cooking, in a large bowl, mix the ricotta, egg white, and pesto together using a plastic spatula.

- Lightly coat an 11 x 7-inch oven-proof baking dish (at least 3 inches deep) with olive oil spray. Lay the slices of yellow squash side by side to create a single layer on the bottom of the dish. Follow with a single layer of zucchini, then a layer of eggplant. Spread a third of the pesto-ricotta mixture on top of the eggplant, followed by a third of the roasted peppers. Top with ½ cup marinara. Repeat this two times. Finish with a layer of marinara.

- Cover with aluminum foil and bake for 30 minutes. Remove the foil and bake for 15 minutes more. Once cooked, let rest on a cooling rack for 10 minutes before slicing and serving.

**PER SERVING:** 348 calories / 21 g fat / 29 g carb / 8 g fiber / 15 g protein

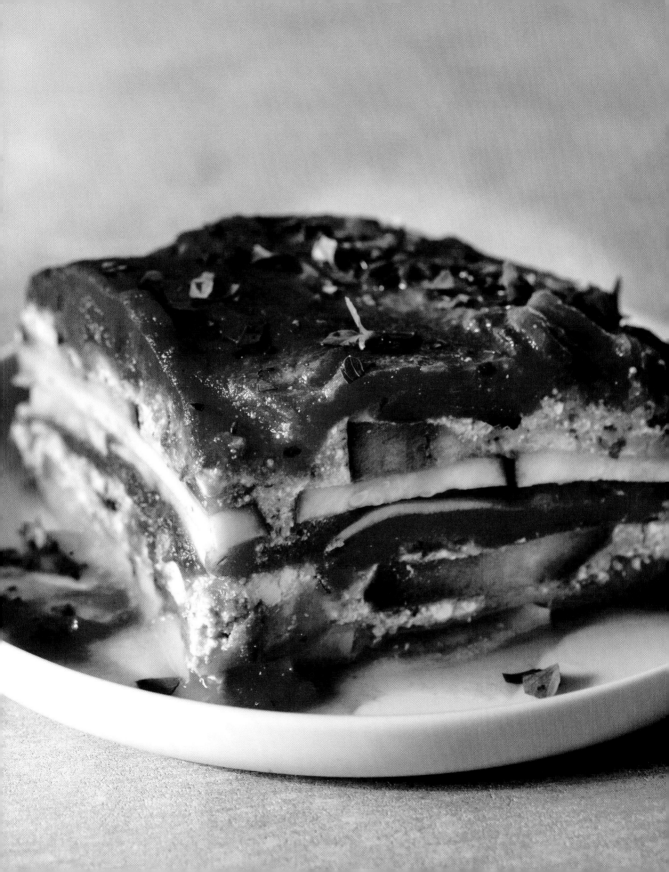

# VEGETABLE FRITTATA with BLUEBERRY ARUGULA SALAD

**SERVES: 4    COOK TIME: 30 MINUTES**

## Frittata

Olive oil spray

8   whole eggs

4   egg whites

1   cup packed chopped fresh spinach

1   cup Salsa (page 245), or store-bought

¼   tsp freshly ground black pepper

¼   tsp kosher salt

## Salad

4   cups baby arugula

½   cup blueberries, rinsed

2   tbsp raw walnuts, toasted in a dry pan over medium heat until fragrant (about 2 minutes), and coarsely chopped

1   large red apple, seeded and sliced into half-moons

2   tbsp Zero Belly Vinaigrette (page 236)

- Preheat the oven to 425°F.

- Lightly coat a 10-inch round baking dish with olive oil spray.

- Whisk together the eggs and egg whites. Add the remaining frittata ingredients and whisk again to combine. Pour into the prepared baking dish and cook, uncovered, for 30 minutes or until the eggs are completely cooked.

- Transfer the frittata to a cooling rack to rest uncovered, for about 5 minutes.

- Combine the salad ingredients in a large bowl and toss to mix.

- Slice the frittata into eight wedges. Divide the salad among four plates and serve with two wedges of frittata.

**PER SERVING:** 229 calories / 13 g fat / 14 g carb / 2 g fiber / 15 g protein

# TURKEY and MUSHROOM QUESADILLAS

**SERVES: 4    COOK TIME: 20 MINUTES**

Olive oil spray

½ **lb lean ground turkey** (at least 93% lean)

½ **cup sliced button mushrooms**

2 **tbsp Mexican Spice Blend** (page 240)

4 **cups mixed greens**

1 **tbsp Zero Belly Vinaigrette** (page 236)

4 **8 to 10-inch gluten-free tortillas**

½ **cup grated cheddar cheese***

½ **cup Salsa** (page 245)

¼ **cup Guacamole** (page 243)

Pre-shredded cheese includes additives like cellulose (derived from wood chips) to prevent the shreds from gumming up. Dodge sawdust and save money by buying block cheese and shredding your own!

**PER SERVING:**
439 calories / 27 g fat /
30 g carb / 5 g fiber /
17 g protein

- Heat a large skillet sprayed with olive oil spray over medium-high heat. Add the ground turkey and use a rubber spatula or a wooden spoon to break up the ground turkey into small pieces. Cook until browned, 3 to 5 minutes. Add the mushrooms and spice mix to the pan and mix well. Continue to cook, stirring often, until the mushrooms are soft. Remove from the heat and, with a slotted spoon, transfer the turkey to a plate covered in paper towels to drain any excess fat.

- Toss together the mixed greens and vinaigrette in a large bowl.

- Place 2 tortillas on a cutting board or clean surface. Divide the cooked turkey mixture evenly between both tortillas. Top each tortilla with ¼ cup shredded cheese and top with another tortilla.

- Spray a large sauté pan with olive oil spray and heat over medium-high heat. Place the quesadilla in the pan. Cook until the tortilla becomes golden brown and crispy, 2 to 3 minutes. Flip the quesadilla in the pan and cook for 2 minutes more, or until browned. Transfer the quesadilla to a cooling rack. Repeat the process for the second quesadilla.

- Cut each quesadilla into quarters. Divide the mixed greens among four plates. Serve with two wedges of quesadilla and a side of 2 tablespoons salsa and 1 tablespoon guacamole.

# BBQ SPICED NUTS

YIELD: 4 CUPS     BAKE TIME: 25 MINUTES

## BBQ SPICED NUTS

1   tsp kosher salt
2   tsp smoked paprika
1   tsp garlic powder
½   tsp dry mustard
½   tsp ground cumin
½   tsp ground ginger
2   egg whites
3   tbsp maple syrup
4   cups raw mixed nuts
    Olive oil spray

## SWEET SPICED NUTS

¾   tsp kosher salt
2   tsp ground cinnamon
1   tsp ground allspice
½   tsp ground clove
½   tsp ground nutmeg
1   tbsp (packed) brown sugar
2   egg whites
3   tbsp maple syrup
4   cups raw mixed nuts
    Olive oil spray

*For both recipes:*

- Preheat the oven to 350°F.

- Mix together the kosher salt, spices, and brown sugar (for Sweet Spiced Nuts) in a small bowl.

- In a large bowl, whisk the egg whites until foamy. Whisk in the maple syrup. Add the nuts and toss to coat. Stir in the spices and mix until evenly coated.

- Spoon the nuts onto a nonstick rimmed baking sheet lightly coated in olive oil spray. Spread evenly.

- Bake for 25 minutes, stirring two or three times throughout, until the nuts are dry and toasted.

- Transfer the baking sheet to a cooling rack to cool. Serve warm or at room temperature.

**PER ¼ CUP:**
182 calories / 14 g fat / 3 g carb /
3 g fiber / 5 g protein

**PER ¼ CUP:**
182 calories / 14 g fat / 3 g carb /
3 g fiber / 5 g protein

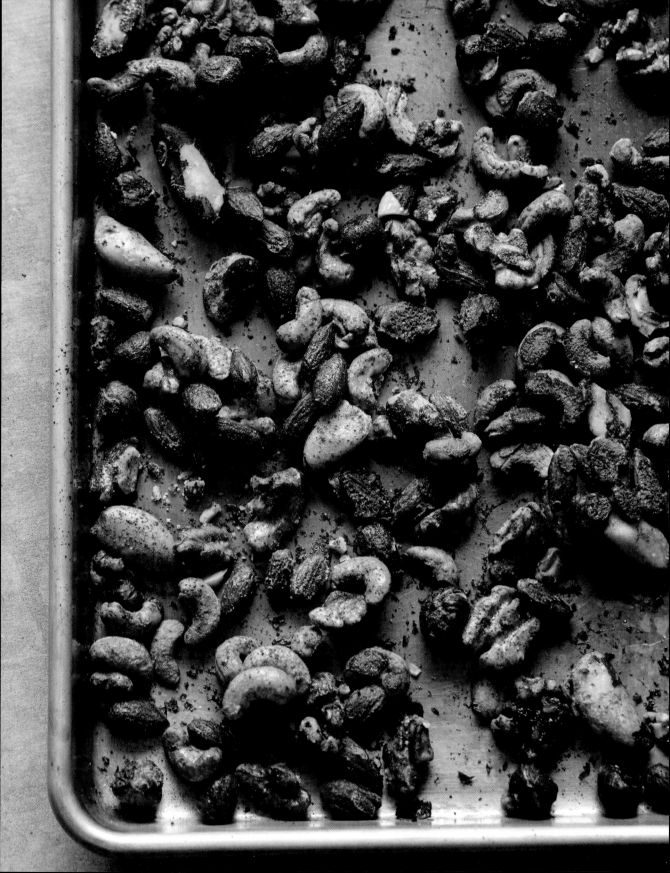

# CHOCOLATE COCONUT POPCORN

SERVES: 4 (ABOUT 8 CUPS TOTAL)   COOK TIME: 5 MINUTES

1 tbsp virgin coconut oil

¼ cup popcorn kernels

2 oz semisweet chocolate (chips or bar, chopped)

½ cup unsweetened flaked coconut

- Melt the coconut oil in a large saucepan (at least 4 quarts) over medium-high heat. Add the popcorn, and cover with a lid. Shake the pot every 5 seconds until the popcorn starts to pop. Once the popcorn starts to pop, shake constantly back and forth until the popping slows to one pop every 2 seconds. Remove from the heat and take off the lid.

- Place the chocolate chips in a small saucepan and melt over low heat, stirring with a small heatproof spatula to ensure that the chocolate does not burn.

- Add half the chocolate and half the flaked coconut to the popcorn and stir. Repeat with the remaining chocolate and flaked coconut and stir for even coverage.

- Serve warm or cooled.

**PER SERVING:** 183 calories / 13 g fat / 17 g carb / 5 g fiber / 5 g protein

# SPICY POPCORN

**SERVES: 4 (ABOUT 8 CUPS TOTAL)** **COOK TIME: 5 MINUTES**

1   **tbsp virgin coconut oil**

¼   **cup popcorn kernels**

1   **tsp smoked paprika**

¼   **tsp ground cinnamon**

¼   **tsp ground cumin**

¼   **tsp garlic powder**

¼   **tsp kosher salt**

**PER SERVING:** 118 calories / 5 g fat / 19 g carb / 3 g fiber / 3 g protein

- Melt the coconut oil in a large saucepan (at least 4 quarts) over medium-high heat. Add the popcorn, and cover with a lid. Shake the pot every 5 seconds until the popcorn starts to pop. Once the popcorn starts to pop, shake constantly back and forth until the popping slows to one pop every 2 seconds. Remove from the heat and take off the lid.

- In a small bowl, mix together the spices and salt. Sprinkle the spice mixture over the cooked popcorn and toss to incorporate.

- Serve warm or cooled.


# KALE CHIPS

**SERVES: 2** **COOK TIME: 20 MINUTES**

1   **head kale,** rinsed and dried well in a salad spinner or on paper towels

   **Olive oil spray**

   **Sea salt**

**PER SERVING:** 80 calories / 1 g fat / 10 g carb / 4 g fiber / 4 g protein

- Preheat the oven to 300°F.

- Place the kale leaves on a rimmed baking sheet (or two) in a single layer, and spray the leaves with olive oil spray. Turn over the leaves and repeat, taking care not to overlap the leaves. Sprinkle very lightly with a pinch of sea salt.

- Bake in the oven for 10 minutes. Turn over the kale and bake for 10 minutes more, or until crispy.

- Transfer the baking sheets to a cooling rack to cool completely.

# DEVILED EGGS

SERVES: 4   COOK TIME: N/A

4   hard-boiled eggs
    (page 250)
2   tbsp Zero Belly
    Mayonnaise (page 242)
1   tbsp relish
1   tbsp Dijon mustard
¼   tsp smoked paprika

- Slice each egg in half lengthwise and scoop the egg yolks into a small mixing bowl. Place the whites on a serving dish.

- Mash the yolks into a crumble with a fork. Stir in the mayonnaise, relish, and mustard. Evenly disperse heaping teaspoons of yolk mixture back into the egg whites. Sprinkle with paprika before serving.

**PER SERVING (2 halves):** 119 calories / 9 g fat / 2 g carb / 1 g fiber / 7 g protein


# AVOCADO WITH CRAB SALAD

SERVES: 4   COOK TIME: N/A

1   avocado, cut in half,
    pit removed
½   lb fresh crabmeat
2   tbsp Salsa,
    strained of juice
    (page 245)
2   tbsp Zero Belly
    Mayonnaise (page 242)
1   lime
    Kosher salt
    A few sprigs fresh cilantro
    (optional)

- Slice the avocado halves in half again, lengthwise, and place on a plate, pit side up.

- In a medium bowl, fold the crabmeat, salsa, and mayonnaise together using a rubber spatula. Spoon heaping spoonfuls of the crab mixture into the avocado "pits."

- Squeeze the lime all over the avocado and the crab, season with a pinch of salt, and garnish with fresh cilantro, if using.

- Serve immediately.

**PER SERVING:** 191 calories / 13 g fat / 5 g carb / 3 g fiber / 14 g protein

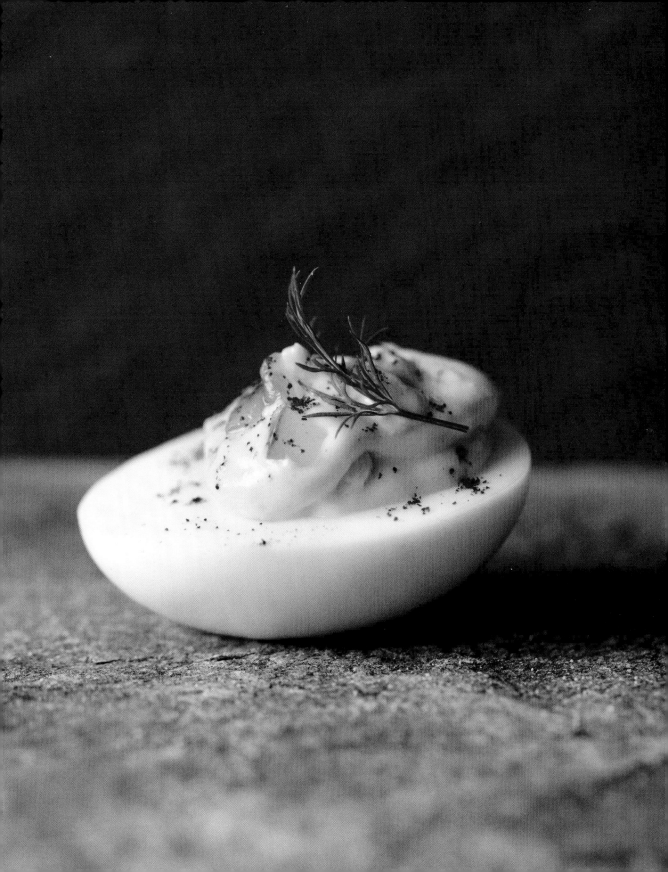

# FRESH FIGS and RICOTTA

SERVES: 4    COOK TIME: N/A

⅓ **cup part-skim ricotta cheese**

3 **tbsp raw Manuka honey**

6 **fresh figs,** quartered

2 **tbsp raw walnuts,** toasted in a dry pan over medium heat until fragrant (about 2 minutes) and coarsely chopped

**Freshly ground black pepper**

- Mix together the ricotta and honey and divide among four small bowls. Top with 6 pieces of fresh fig. Garnish with the toasted walnuts and a pinch of pepper.

**PER SERVING:** 126 calories / 4 g fat / 20 g carb / 3 g fiber / 4 g protein

# RED FRUITS with HONEY-NUT DIP

SERVES: 4    COOK TIME: N/A

½ **cup natural, no-salt-added peanut butter or almond butter**

½ **cup light coconut milk**

1 **tbsp raw Manuka honey**

1 **peach,** skin on, cut into wedges

1 **apple,** skin on, cut into wedges

1 **cup strawberries**

- Place the nut butter, coconut milk, and honey in the bowl of a food processor and puree until smooth.

- Arrange the fruit on a platter and serve family style with a small bowl of honey-nut dip.

**PER SERVING:** 203 calories / 13 g fat / 18 g carb / 4 g fiber / 7 g protein

# BANANAS with NUTTY HONEY-CINNAMON DIP

SERVES: 4    COOK TIME: N/A

½  cup natural, no-salt-added peanut butter or almond butter

½  cup light coconut milk

1  tbsp raw Manuka honey

1  tsp ground cinnamon

½  tsp vanilla extract

2  large bananas, peeled and cut into 1-inch slices

- Place the nut butter, coconut milk, honey, cinnamon, and vanilla in the bowl of a food processor and puree until smooth.

- Arrange the banana chunks on a plate and serve family style with a small bowl of nutty honey-cinnamon dip.

**PER SERVING:** 219 calories / 13 g fat / 22 g carb / 4 g fiber / 7 g protein

# ZERO BELLY GRANOLA

YIELD: 6 CUPS    COOK TIME: 25 MINUTES

4 **cups rolled oats**

¼ **cup raw walnuts,** chopped

¼ **cup raw pecans,** chopped

⅓ **cup pistachios,** shelled

⅓ **cup dried tart cherries,** chopped

¼ **cup maple syrup**

2 **tbsp extra-virgin olive oil**

2 **egg whites**

½ **tsp ground cinnamon**

¼ **tsp kosher salt**

- Preheat the oven to 325°F.

- Mix the oats, walnuts, pecans, pistachios, and cherries together in a large bowl.

- In another bowl, whisk together the maple syrup, olive oil, egg whites, cinnamon, and kosher salt. Pour over the oats and nuts and stir to combine.

- Spread the mixture evenly on two nonstick rimmed baking sheets.

- Bake in the oven for 25 minutes, or until golden. Stir after 10 minutes for an even color and to ensure that the granola cooks evenly.

- Transfer to a cooling rack to cool.

**PER ½ CUP:** 201 calories / 8 g fat / 30 g carb / 5 g fiber / 7 g protein

# CHICKEN SATAY
# with PEANUT SAUCE

**SERVES: 4** | **COOK TIME: 10 MINUTES**

### Marinade

- **1  clove garlic**
- **1  tbsp low-sodium tamari**
- **1  ½-inch piece of fresh ginger,** peeled
- **1  tbsp extra-virgin olive oil**

- **8  oz skinless, boneless chicken breast,** diced into ½-inch cubes

### Peanut Sauce

- **2  tbsp natural, no-salt-added peanut butter**
- **¼  cup light coconut milk**
- **½  tsp tamari**
- **½  tsp fresh lime juice**
- **½  tsp chili flakes** (optional)

### Special Equipment

- **8  wooden skewers,** soaked in water for 10 minutes to prevent burning

- Blend the marinade ingredients in the bowl of a food processor. Combine the cubed chicken and marinade in a bowl and allow to marinate for 10 minutes.

- Use a slotted spoon or tongs to transfer the marinated chicken to a plate lined with paper towels. Slide the chicken cubes onto the soaked wooden skewers.

- Heat an outdoor grill or grill pan over medium heat.

- Place the skewers on the grill and cook for 4 minutes. Flip and cook for 4 minutes more.

- While the skewers are cooking, place all of the ingredients for the peanut sauce in the bowl of a food processor and puree until smooth.

- Serve the grilled skewers hot with a small bowl of peanut sauce.

**PER SERVING:** 185 calories / 10 g fat / 3 g carb / 2 g fiber / 20 g protein

# ARTICHOKES with GARLIC LEMON DIPPING SAUCE

**SERVES: 4   COOK TIME: 30 MINUTES**

**Salt**

2 **large artichokes,**
washed in cold water

**Kosher salt**

*Garlic Lemon Dipping Sauce*

¼ **cup Zero Belly Mayonnaise**
(page 242)

**Juice of ½ lemon**

4 **cloves garlic,**
minced

1 **tsp kosher salt**

- Fill a large pot of water halfway with water. Salt the water as you would for pasta and bring to a boil.

- Prepare the artichokes by trimming the stems so only 1 inch of stem remains. Tear off any small or loose leaves from the artichoke with your fingers.

- Submerge the trimmed artichokes in the salted boiling water and reduce to a slow simmer. Placing a lid that's smaller than the pot directly atop the artichokes will ensure that they stay submerged. Cook until tender, about 30 minutes.

- While the artichokes are cooking, combine the ingredients for the dipping sauce in a small bowl and mix well.

- After the artichokes have cooked for about 30 minutes, use a small knife to poke the stems; they should be tender but not mushy. Place the cooked artichokes upside down in a colander to drain.

- Serve warm with the sauce.

**PER SERVING:** 124 calories / 10 g fat / 8 g carb / 4 g fiber / 2 g protein

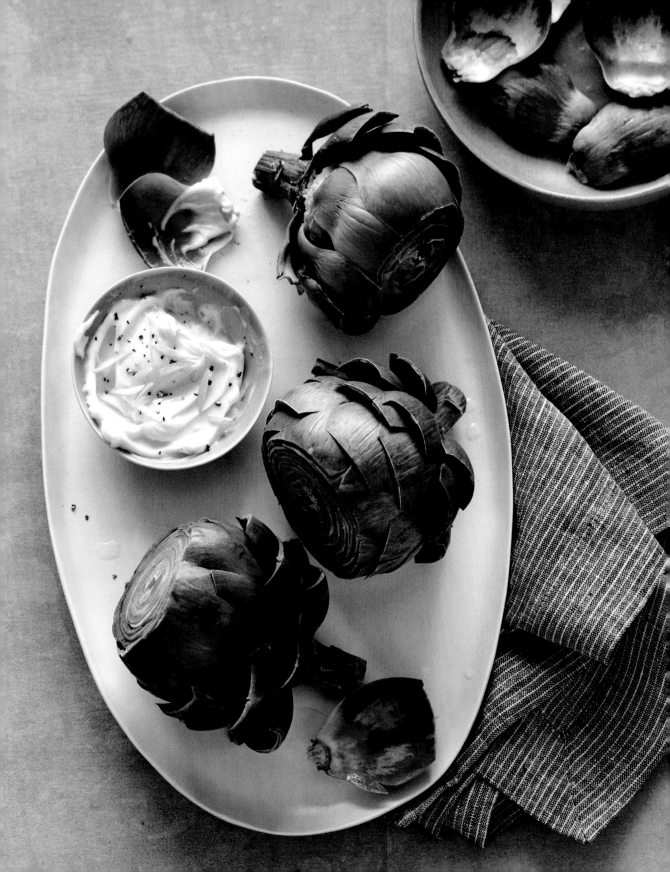

# CRUDITÉS and DIPS

SERVES: 4　COOK TIME: N/A

### CRUDITÉS and HUMMUS

- **2 to 3 large carrots,** peeled and sliced into sticks, about 4 inches long and ½ inch thick

- **8 stalks celery,** sliced into sticks, about 4 inches long and ½ inch thick

- **1½ cups cherry or grape tomatoes,** left whole

- **1½ cups thick slices English cucumber**

- **1 cup Hummus** (page 244)

### CRUDITÉS and ROASTED RED PEPPER DIP

- **1½ cups fennel,** cut into ¼-inch-thick sticks, blanched*

- **1 bunch green asparagus** (about 12 spears), white part of stem removed, blanched*

- **1½ cups green beans,** blanched*

- **1½ cups jicama,** peeled and cut into ½-inch-thick sticks

- **1 cup Roasted Red Pepper Dip** (page 245)

### CRUDITÉS and GREEN GODDESS DRESSING

- **1½ cups radishes,** sliced in half if large

- **1½ cups raw cauliflower florets,** large florets cut in half

- **1½ cups cherry or grape tomatoes,** left whole

- **1½ cups thick slices of English cucumber**

- **1 cup Green Goddess Dressing** (page 244)

*For all recipes:*

- Arrange the crudités on a platter and serve family style with a small bowl of dip.

To blanch vegetables, bring a large pot of water to a boil. Meanwhile, fill a large bowl with ice and cold water. Drop the vegetables into the boiling water for 1 to 2 minutes. Use a slotted spoon to transfer the vegetables from the hot water directly to the ice bath to cool. Drain them in a colander and transfer to a plate covered with paper towel to dry completely.

**PER SERVING:** 108 calories / 3 g fat / 18 g carb / 6 g fiber / 4 g protein

**PER SERVING:** 129 calories / 9 g fat / 11 g carb / 4 g fiber / 4 g protein

**PER SERVING:** 146 calories / 10 g fat / 12 g carb / 6 g fiber / 4 g protein

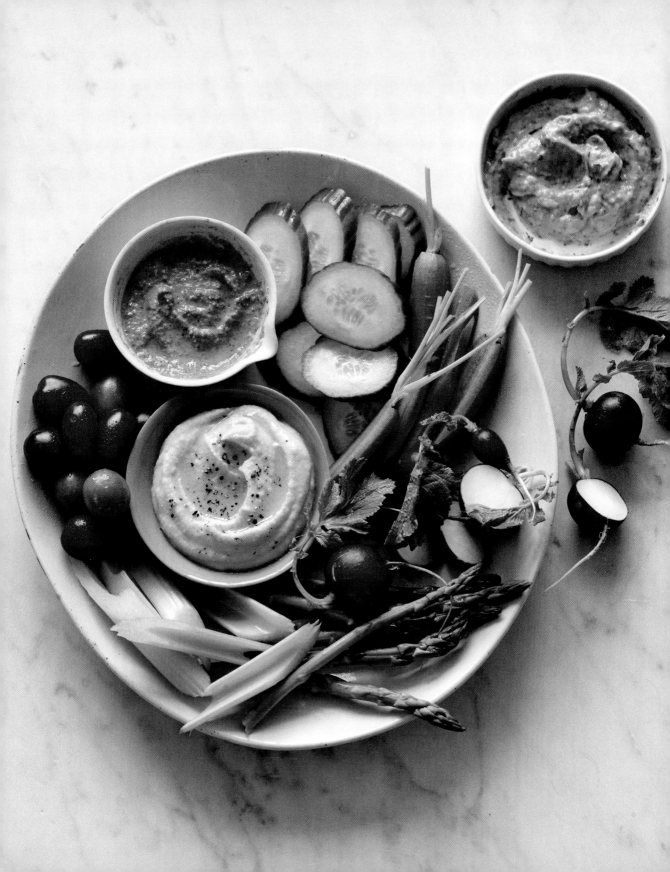

# SMOKED SALMON and CUCUMBER ROUNDS with HERBED MAYONNAISE

**SERVES: 4    COOK TIME: N/A**

*Herbed Mayonnaise*

- **3 tbsp Zero Belly Mayonnaise** (page 242)

- **1 tsp chopped fresh dill or tarragon**

- **Juice of ½ lemon**


- **1 English cucumber,** skin on, sliced into ¼-inch-thick disks

- **4 oz smoked Atlantic salmon**

- Whisk together the herbed mayonnaise ingredients in a small bowl and set aside.

- Lay the cucumber rounds on a plate. Tear off pieces of the salmon, about the size of a half-dollar. Pinch the salmon together to make a flowerlike shape. Place on the cucumber rounds.

- Spoon a small amount of herbed mayonnaise on top of the bites. Serve immediately.

**PER SERVING:** 112 calories / 9 g fat / 3 g carb / 2 g fiber / 6 g protein

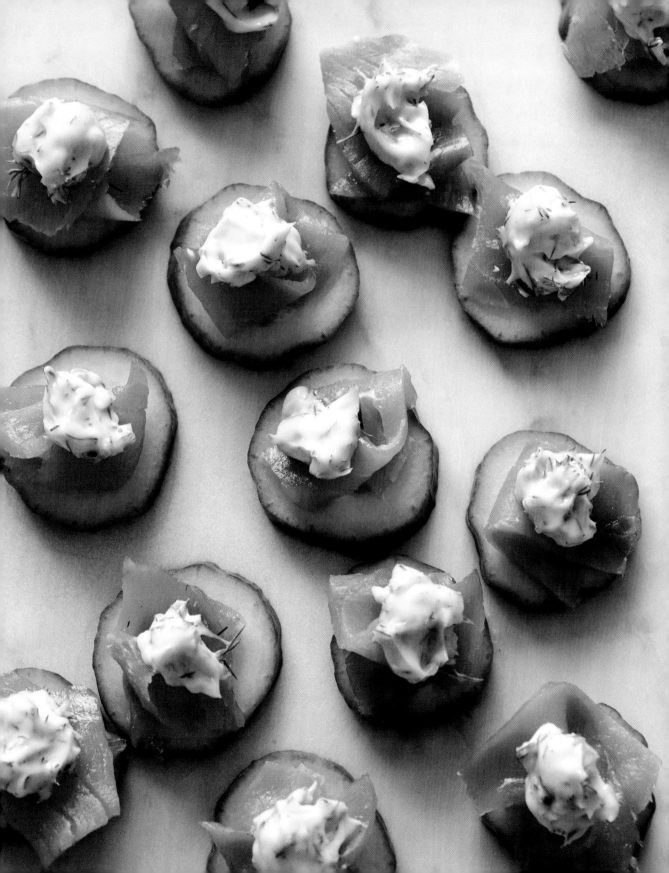

# BUFFALO CHICKEN SKEWERS

SERVES: 4    COOK TIME: 10 MINUTES

8  **oz skinless, boneless chicken breasts,** diced into ½-inch pieces

½  **cup Red-Hot Buffalo Dressing** (page 237)

8  **stalks celery,** halved (or cut into thirds, depending on size)

*Special Equipment*

8  **wooden skewers,** soaked in water for 10 minutes to prevent burning

- Combine the cubed chicken and ¼ cup Red Hot Buffalo Dressing in a bowl and allow to marinate for 10 minutes.

- Use a slotted spoon or tongs to transfer the marinated chicken to a plate lined with paper towels. Slide the chicken cubes onto the soaked wooden skewers, eight total.

- Heat an outdoor grill or grill pan over medium heat.

- Place the skewers on the grill and cook for 4 minutes. Flip and cook for 4 minutes more.

- Place the remaining ¼ cup of Red Hot Buffalo Dressing in a small bowl. Serve alongside the hot grilled skewers and celery sticks.

**PER SERVING:** 192 calories / 16 g fat / 0 g carb / 2 g fiber / 11 g protein

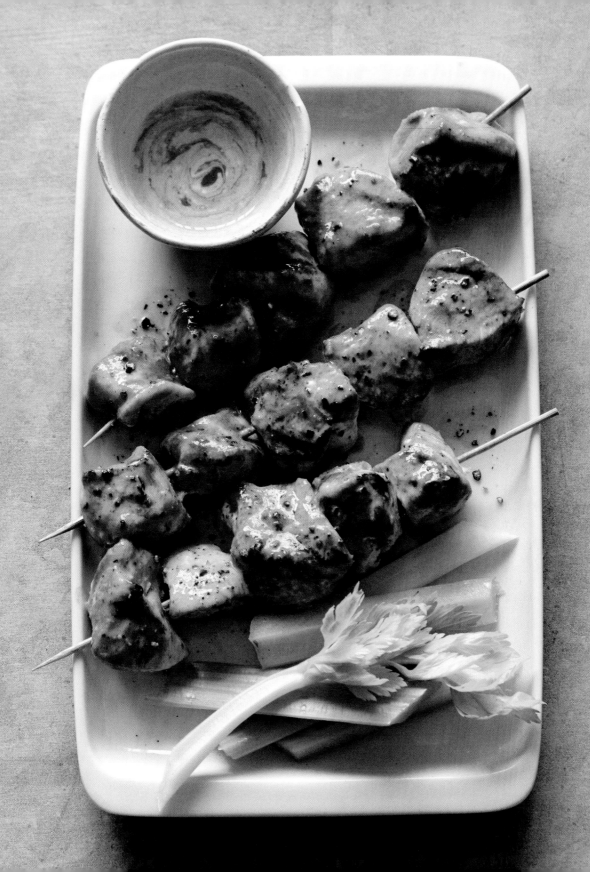

# CHAPTER EIGHT

# ZERO BELLY DESSERTS

Prepare to Revel in the Taste Sensations
of Pure, Indulgent Desserts That Excite Your
Taste Buds—and Flatten Your Tummy

Dessert isn't evil.

After all, it was the simple, healthy apple that got Adam and Eve chased out of paradise, not the apple pie. And while most diet gurus unfairly malign dessert as a girth-promoting serving of sin, it ought to be a well-deserved, nutritious nightcap that actually helps you achieve your weight-loss goals. In fact, according to a Tufts University study, dieters who give in to cravings are more successful than those who don't. The reason: Once you make "watching what you eat" feel less onerous, it becomes easier to stick to your eating plan.

Fortunately, these recipes watch what you eat for you, so you can be sure you're topping off your day with decadent helpings of foods that are actually working for you. Each of these desserts has fiber, protein, and healthy fat—and that makes them perfect cappers for a **ZERO BELLY** day.

# ANGEL FOOD CAKE with WHIPPED COCONUT CREAM and MIXED BERRIES

**SERVES: 12**  **COOK TIME: 45 MINUTES**

| | |
|---|---|
| 12 | egg whites |
| 1½ | cups granulated sugar |
| 1 | cup gluten-free all-purpose flour (like Bob's Red Mill) |
| 1 | tsp cream of tartar |
| 2 | tsp vanilla extract |
| ¼ | tsp kosher salt |
| 1 | cup Whipped Coconut Cream (page 188) |
| 2 | cups fresh mixed berries |

- Place the egg whites in a large bowl. Cover with plastic wrap and let sit at room temperature for 1 hour.

- Preheat the oven to 350°F.

- Sift ¾ cup granulated sugar and the gluten-free flour together in a large bowl.

- Place the egg whites and the cream of tartar in the bowl of a stand mixer or hand mixer. Use a whip attachment to whip the egg whites until foamy.

- While the mixer is running, add 1 tablespoon of the remaining granulated sugar at a time until all of the sugar is incorporated. Add the vanilla and salt to the whipped egg whites and whip to stiff peaks. Do not overwhip.

- Very carefully fold in the sifted dry ingredients, ½ cup at a time, with a rubber spatula.

- Scoop the batter into an ungreased 10-inch Bundt pan.

- Bake for 45 minutes, or until very light golden brown. Transfer to a cooling rack and allow to cool for at least 30 minutes.

- Run a small knife along the edges of the cake to free it from the pan. Flip the pan over onto a large plate. Remove the pan.

- Garnish with Whipped Coconut Cream and fresh berries. Cut into slices and serve.

**PER SERVING:** 184 calories / 3 g fat / 34 g carb / 2 g fiber / 5 g protein

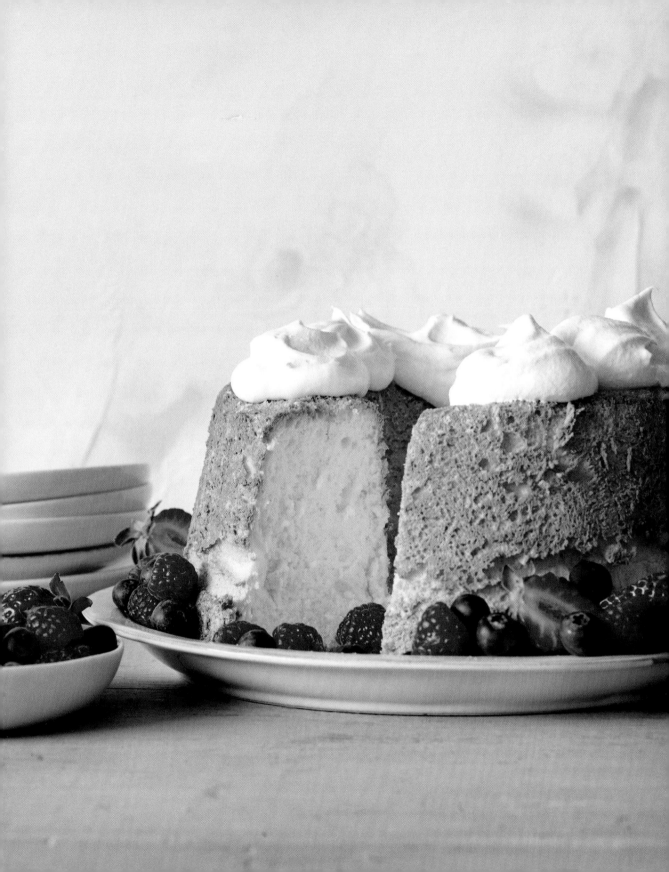

# CHOCOLATE BARK

**SERVES: 10   COOK TIME: 5 MINUTES**

**10** **oz semisweet chocolate chips**

**¼** **cup dried tart cherries**

**¼** **cup raw pepitas,** toasted in a dry pan over medium heat until fragrant (about 2 minutes) and cooled

**¼** **cup raw almonds,** toasted in a dry pan over medium heat until fragrant (about 2 minutes), cooled, and coarsely chopped

- Preheat the oven to 350°F.

- Line a rimmed baking sheet with parchment paper. Pour the chocolate chips onto the parchment paper and spread to form a rectangle, about 8 x 8 inches.

- Bake the chocolate chips in the oven for 2 to 3 minutes, just until they start to melt.

- Transfer the baking sheet to a cooling rack and use an offset spatula to spread the melted chocolate into a smooth, even rectangle. While the chocolate is still hot, evenly sprinkle with the dried cherries, toasted pepitas, and toasted almonds. Transfer the parchment paper to a plate and refrigerate for at least 30 minutes. Break the bark into small pieces and serve.

**PER SERVING:** 190 calories / 12 g fat / 22 g carb / 2 g fiber / 3 g protein

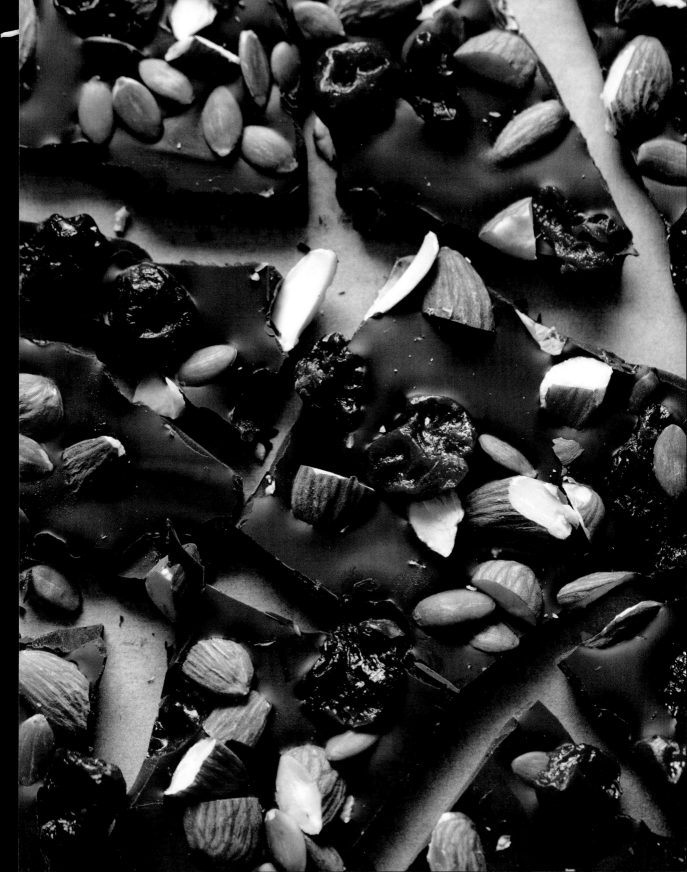

# WHIPPED COCONUT CREAM

1  **14-oz can full-fat, unsweetened coconut milk,** refrigerated for at least 1 hour

¼  **tsp vanilla extract**

- Open the cold can of coconut milk. There will be a thick layer of "cream" on top and the water on the bottom. Carefully scoop out the cream with a spoon and place in a bowl.

- With a hand blender or a stand mixer fixed with a whisk attachment, whip the coconut milk for 3 to 4 minutes, until it is fluffy and resembles whipped cream. Whisk in the vanilla.

- Refrigerate until ready to use.

**PER ¼ CUP:** 116 calories / 12 g fat / 2 g carb / 0 g fiber / 1 g protein

# CHOCOLATE ALMOND PROTEIN TRUFFLES

YIELD: 12 TRUFFLES    COOK TIME: N/A

- ½ **cup natural, no-salt-added almond butter**
- 2 **tbsp raw Manuka honey**
- ⅔ **cup chocolate plant-based protein powder**
- ⅛ **tsp kosher salt**
- ¼ **cup raw almonds,** dry roasted in a pan over medium heat until fragrant (about 2 minutes) and finely chopped

- Mix together the almond butter, honey, protein powder, and salt in a bowl.

- Roll the truffle mixture into twelve 1-inch balls. Roll in the toasted almonds.

- Place in the fridge for 1 hour and serve cold.

**PER TRUFFLE:** 122 calories / 7 g fat / 7 g carb / 2 g fiber / 10 g protein

# APPLE CRUMBLE

**SERVES: 8   COOK TIME: 1 HOUR 30 MINUTES**

Olive oil spray

6 **red apples,** skin on, diced into ½-inch cubes

**Zest and juice of 1 orange**

¼ **cup (packed) brown sugar**

1 **tsp ground cinnamon**

¼ **tsp ground nutmeg**

*Crumble Topping*

¾ **cup rolled oats,** ground to a flour in the bowl of a food processor

¼ **cup (packed) brown sugar**

¼ **cup coconut oil,** melted

- Preheat the oven to 350°F.

- Spray a 9 x 9-inch pan or baking dish with olive oil spray.

- Combine the diced apples with the orange juice, orange zest, brown sugar, cinnamon, and nutmeg. Mix well and spread evenly in the prepared baking dish.

- Place the crumble topping ingredients in a separate bowl and mix with your hands, pinching it together into clumps.

- Evenly spread the crumble topping on the apples.

- Cover with aluminum foil and bake for 30 minutes. Remove the foil and bake for 45 minutes more, until golden brown.

- Transfer to a cooling rack and let cool for 5 minutes. Serve warm or at room temperature.

**PER SERVING:** 234 calories / 9 g fat / 39 g carb / 2 g fiber / 5 g protein

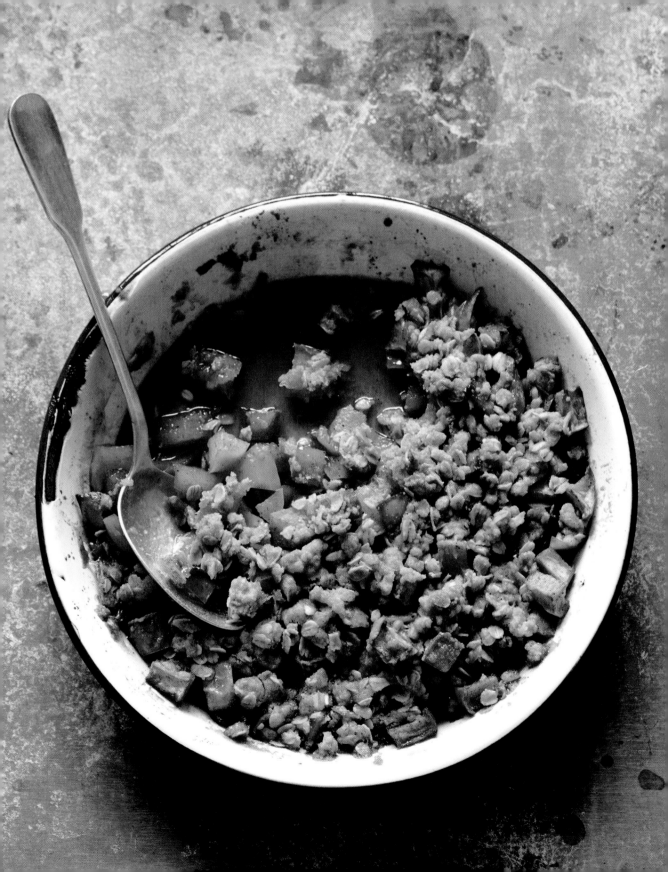

# DESSERT PIZZA with WHIPPED COCONUT CREAM and SUMMER BERRIES

SERVES: 4    COOK TIME: 10 MINUTES

2   gluten-free tortillas
    Olive oil spray
½   cup Whipped
    Coconut Cream
    (page 188)
¼   cup fresh blueberries
¼   cup fresh raspberries
¼   cup fresh blackberries
¼   cup fresh strawberries,
    quartered
2   tbsp coarsely chopped
    fresh mint

- Preheat the oven to 350°F.

- Place the tortillas on a rimmed baking sheet and lightly spray each side with olive oil spray. Bake for 3 to 5 minutes, until crispy. Transfer to a cooling rack or plate to cool completely.

- Divide the Whipped Coconut Cream between the two tortillas and spread to cover.

- Place half of the blueberries in the center of the whipped cream, followed by a ring of half the raspberries, half the blackberries, and then half the strawberries. Repeat with the second tortilla.

- Garnish the pizzas with chopped mint, slice into wedges, and serve immediately.

PER SERVING: 167 calories / 8 g fat / 23 g carb / 9 g fiber / 2 g protein

# BANANA CUPCAKES

YIELD: 12 CUPCAKES    COOK TIME: 25 MINUTES

1½ cups gluten-free all-purpose flour (like Bob's Red Mill)

2 tsp baking powder

½ tsp kosher salt

3 large eggs

⅓ cup (packed) light brown sugar

⅓ cup coconut oil, melted

1½ tsp vanilla extract

1 tbsp fresh lemon juice

¼ cup unsweetened almond milk

¼ cup natural, no-salt-added peanut butter or almond butter

3 ripe bananas, mashed

½ cup semisweet chocolate chips

- Preheat the oven to 350°F.

- Line a standard 12-hole muffin tin with cupcake liners.

- In a large bowl, mix together the flour, baking powder, and salt.

- In another large bowl, whisk together the eggs, brown sugar, coconut oil, vanilla, lemon juice, almond milk, and nut butter until smooth.

- Add the dry ingredients to the wet ingredients and mix until just incorporated. Fold in the bananas and chocolate chips. Do not overmix.

- Divide the mixture among the 12 muffin cups and bake for 25 minutes, or until a toothpick inserted in the center of a muffin comes out clean.

- Transfer to a cooling rack and allow to cool completely. Serve at room temperature.

**PER CUPCAKE:** 254 calories / 13 g fat / 31 g carb / 3 g fiber / 6 g protein

# CARROT CAKE CUPCAKES

YIELD: 12 CUPCAKES    COOK TIME: 25 MINUTES

- 1⅓ cup gluten-free all-purpose flour (like Bob's Red Mill)
- ½ tsp baking soda
- ½ tsp kosher salt
- 2 tsp ground cinnamon
- 1 tsp ground ginger
- ½ tsp ground nutmeg
- 1 large egg
- 1 large egg white
- ⅓ cup coconut oil, melted
- ½ cup (packed) light brown sugar
- 1 tsp vanilla extract
- ½ cup grated carrots
- 1 cup Whipped Coconut Cream (page 188)

- Preheat the oven to 350°F.

- Line a standard 12-hole muffin tin with cupcake liners.

- Mix together the flour, baking soda, salt, cinnamon, ginger, and nutmeg. Set aside.

- In another large bowl, mix together the egg, egg white, coconut oil, brown sugar, and vanilla.

- Add the dry ingredients to the wet ingredients and mix to incorporate. Do not overmix. Fold in the carrots.

- Spoon the batter into the 12 cupcake liners and bake for 20 minutes, or until a toothpick inserted in the center of a muffin comes out clean.

- While the cupcakes are baking, prepare the Whipped Coconut Cream.

- Transfer the cupcakes to a cooling rack and allow to cool completely.

- Top the cooled cupcakes with a dollop of Whipped Coconut Cream. Serve immediately.

**PER CUPCAKE:** 176 calories / 10 g fat / 20 g carb / 2 g fiber / 3 g protein

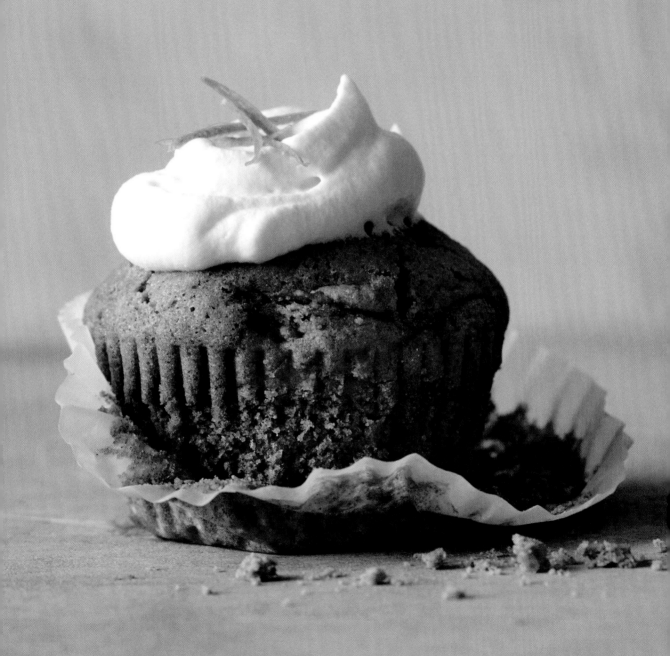

# RASPBERRY POACHED PEARS

SERVES: 4    COOK TIME: 40 MINUTES

1   **cup raspberries**
    (fresh or frozen)

1   **qt water**

¼   **cup raw Manuka honey**

1   **cinnamon stick**

3   **cloves**
    (optional)

2   **Bosc pears,**
    peeled, halved, and cored

¼   **cup raw flaked almonds,**
    toasted in a dry pan
    over medium heat
    until fragrant (about
    2 minutes)

¼   **cup fresh raspberries**

- Place the raspberries, water, and honey in the bowl of a food processor and puree until smooth. Transfer the mixture to a medium saucepan. Add the puree, cinnamon stick, and cloves to the saucepan and stir to incorporate.

- Add the pear halves to the saucepan and bring to a low simmer over medium heat. Cover with a lid and cook for about 35 minutes. Flip the pears over one or two times while cooking. Once the pears are fork tender, remove the pan from heat and allow the pears to cool in the poaching liquid for up to 24 hours in advance of serving.

- Place each pear half on a dessert plate or in a bowl and top with ¼ cup of the poaching liquid. Garnish with 1 tablespoon flaked almonds and a few fresh raspberries.

**PER SERVING:** 141 calories / 0 g fat / 37 g carb / 5 g fiber / 2 g protein

# GRILLED PEACHES with COCONUT WHIPPED CREAM and TOASTED ALMONDS

SERVES: 4    COOK TIME: 10 MINUTES

**2**  **ripe but firm peaches or nectarines,** skin on, halved, and pits removed

**2**  **tbsp raw Manuka honey**

**½**  **cup Whipped Coconut Cream** (page 188)

**¼**  **cup raw flaked almonds,** toasted in a dry pan over medium heat until fragrant (about 2 minutes)

- Preheat an outdoor grill or grill pan over medium heat.

- Place the fruit flesh-side down on the grill and leave to grill, undisturbed, for 2 minutes. Quarter-turn the fruit on the same side, and leave to grill, undisturbed, for 2 minutes more.

- Flip the fruit and repeat: Grill the fruit for 2 minutes; quarter-turn and allow to grill for 2 minutes more.

- Transfer each grilled fruit half to a plate and drizzle each with ½ tablespoon honey. Top each fruit half with 2 tablespoons Whipped Coconut Cream and 1 tablespoon toasted almonds. Serve immediately.

**PER SERVING:** 166 calories / 9 g fat / 16 g carb / 2 g fiber / 3 g protein

# FLOURLESS CHOCOLATE CAKE

SERVES: 8    COOK TIME: 25 MINUTES

Olive oil spray

6    oz semisweet chocolate
     (chips or bar)

¼    cup maple syrup

½    cup granulated sugar

3    large eggs

½    cup unsweetened
     cocoa powder
     (non-alkalized)

1    tsp vanilla extract

¼    tsp kosher salt

     Fresh berries for garnish

- Preheat the oven to 350°F.

- Lightly spray a 7-inch tart pan with a removable bottom, or a 7- or 8-inch springform pan with olive oil spray. Line the bottom of the pan with parchment paper and spray the paper.

- Melt the chocolate in a small saucepan over low heat together with the maple syrup. Once melted, add the sugar and stir until dissolved, about 2 minutes.

- Take the saucepan off the heat and whisk in the eggs one at a time.

- Sift the cocoa powder with a sieve and whisk into the egg and chocolate mixture. Make sure there are no lumps. Add the vanilla and the salt and mix well.

- Pour the batter into the prepared pan and bake for 25 minutes or until firm to the touch.

- Transfer the cake pan to a cooling rack to rest for at least 5 minutes before slicing.

- Cut the cake into 8 slices, garnish with fresh berries, and serve warm or at room temperature.

**PER SERVING:** 220 calories / 9 g fat / 37 g carb / 2 g fiber / 5 g protein

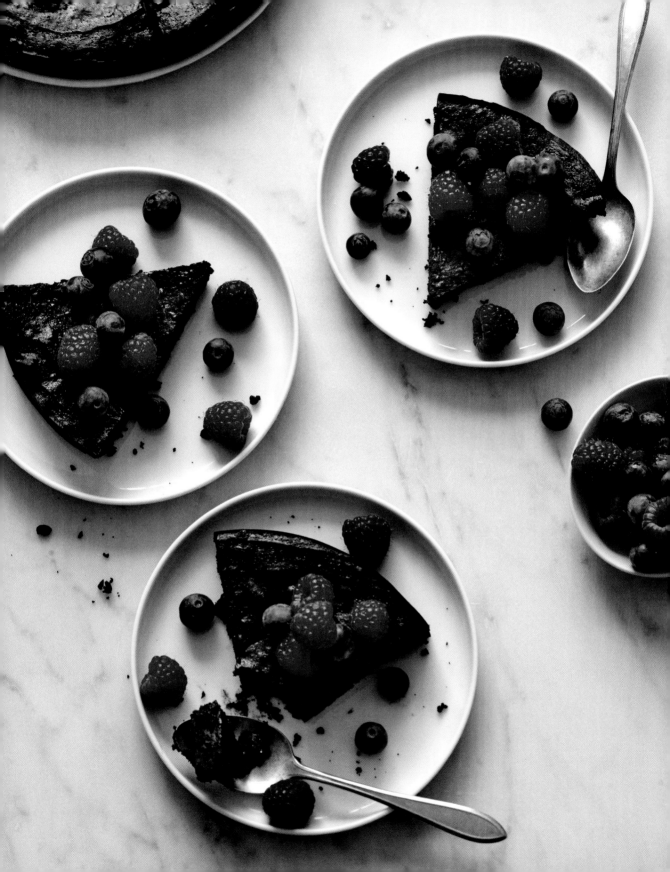

# BROWN RICE CRISPY TREATS

YIELD: 12 BARS    COOK TIME: 10 MINUTES

Olive oil spray

4 cups crispy brown rice cereal

½ cup natural, no-salt-added almond butter

½ cup maple syrup or agave

1 tbsp virgin coconut oil

¼ cup raw almonds, toasted in a dry pan over medium heat until fragrant (about 2 minutes) and coarsely chopped

¼ cup semisweet chocolate chips

- Line a 9 x 9-inch baking dish with parchment paper and spray well with olive oil spray.

- Place the cereal in a large bowl.

- Melt together the almond butter, maple syrup, and coconut oil in a small saucepan over low heat. Use a heatproof spatula or spoon to mix until smooth.

- Pour the hot almond butter mixture over the crispy cereal and use a spatula to mix well. Add the almonds and mix to incorporate.

- Scoop the cereal mixture into the lined baking dish and use your hands to press the mixture evenly in the dish. Sprinkle with chocolate chips and use your hands to lightly press the chocolate into the cereal.

- Refrigerate for at least 2 hours.

- Use a serrated knife to slice into 12 bars. Serve at room temperature.

PER SERVING: 164 calories / 9 g fat / 19 g carb / 3 g fiber / 3 g protein

# CHOCOLATE-DIPPED BANANA POPS

SERVES: 4    COOK TIME: N/A

**2** **ripe bananas**

**5** **oz semisweet chocolate**
(chips or bar, chopped)

¼ **cup raw walnuts,**
toasted in a dry pan
over medium heat
until fragrant
(about 2 minutes)
and coarsely chopped

*Special Equipment*

**4** **wooden craft or
popsicle sticks**

- Line a rimmed baking sheet with parchment paper.

- Peel and cut the bananas in half crosswise and insert a popsicle stick into each half. Place on the prepared baking sheet, and place in the freezer for 30 minutes.

- While the bananas are freezing, place the chocolate in a microwave-safe bowl. Microwave until melted. Stir every 30 seconds.

- Place the chopped walnuts on a plate.

- Dip the frozen bananas in the chocolate, turning them to coat, and then immediately roll them in the chopped walnuts. Return the banana pops to the lined baking sheet, and return to the freezer for at least 45 minutes.

**PER SERVING:** 288 calories / 15 g fat / 40 g carb / 4 g fiber / 2 g protein

# ORANGE DREAMSICLES

YIELD: 8 POPSICLES | COOK TIME: N/A

2 **cups fresh orange juice**
(about 9 large
navel oranges)

1 **large navel orange,**
peeled and segmented

1 **cup light coconut milk**

*Special Equipment*
**Popsicle mold or 8 paper
cups and 8 wooden craft
or popsicle sticks**

- Place the orange juice, orange segments, and coconut milk in a blender and puree until smooth.

- Pour into 8 popsicle molds or paper cups.

- Freeze for 3 hours or until solid. If using paper cups, pull the popsicles out of the freezer after 1½ hours and insert the wooden craft sticks. Continue to freeze until solid.

**PER POPSICLE:** 55 calories / 2 g fat / 9 g carb / 2 g fiber / 1 g protein

# PEANUT BUTTER CHOCOLATE TRUFFLES

YIELD: 20 TRUFFLES   COOK TIME: N/A

**6** oz semisweet chocolate
(chips or bar, chopped)

**¼** cup unsweetened
almond milk

**½** cup natural, no-salt-
added peanut butter
(creamy or crunchy)

- Place the chocolate and the almond milk in a microwave-safe bowl and microwave until melted. Stir every 30 seconds.

- Once melted, whisk in the peanut butter until smooth.

- Cover with plastic wrap and chill in the fridge until firm—at least 3 hours or overnight.

- Use a spoon to scoop large marble-size truffles from the mixture and roll into balls, for about 20 truffles total. Transfer to a tray covered in wax paper and chill in the fridge until firm, about 1 hour.

- Serve cold.

- Store leftovers in a BPA-free container in the fridge for up to 1 week.

**PER TRUFFLE:** 83 calories / 4 g fat / 9 g carb / 2 g fiber / 3 g protein

# RED FRUIT SALAD

SERVES: 4    COOK TIME: N/A

**1 lb fresh strawberries,** quartered

**6 oz fresh raspberries** (1 pint)

**6 oz fresh red plums** (about 3), pits removed and cut into bite-size pieces

**6 oz fresh tart red cherries** (about 2 cups with pits), sliced in half and pits removed

**½ cup fresh pomegranate seeds**

**2 tbsp coarsely chopped fresh mint leaves**

**1 red apple,** skin on, cut into bite-size pieces

**Juice of 1 large orange**

- Place all of the ingredients in a large bowl and toss to combine.

**PER SERVING:** 140 calories / 1 g fat / 30 g carb / 8 g fiber / 4 g protein

# BLACK FOREST COOKIES

YIELD: 24 COOKIES    COOK TIME: 12 MINUTES

**Olive oil spray**

2¼  **cups finely ground almond meal/flour**

¼  **cup unsweetened cocoa powder** (non-alkalized)

½  **tsp baking soda**

½  **cup coconut oil,** melted

½  **cup (packed) light brown sugar**

2  **large eggs**

¾  **cup semisweet chocolate chips**

½  **cup dried tart cherries,** coarsely chopped

- Preheat the oven to 350°F.

- Line 2 rimmed baking sheets with parchment paper and spray with olive oil spray.

- In a large bowl, mix together the almond meal/flour, cocoa powder, and baking soda.

- In another large bowl, whisk together the coconut oil, light brown sugar, and eggs.

- Add the dry ingredients to the wet ingredients and mix to incorporate. Mix in the chocolate chips and dried cherries.

- Use a spoon to scoop out 2 table-spoons of cookie dough onto the baking sheets, leaving about 2 inches between each scoop.

- Bake for 12 minutes. Let the cookies sit for 2 minutes before transferring to a cooling rack to cool.

**PER SERVING:** 211 calories / 17 g fat / 14 g carb / 3 g fiber / 3 g protein

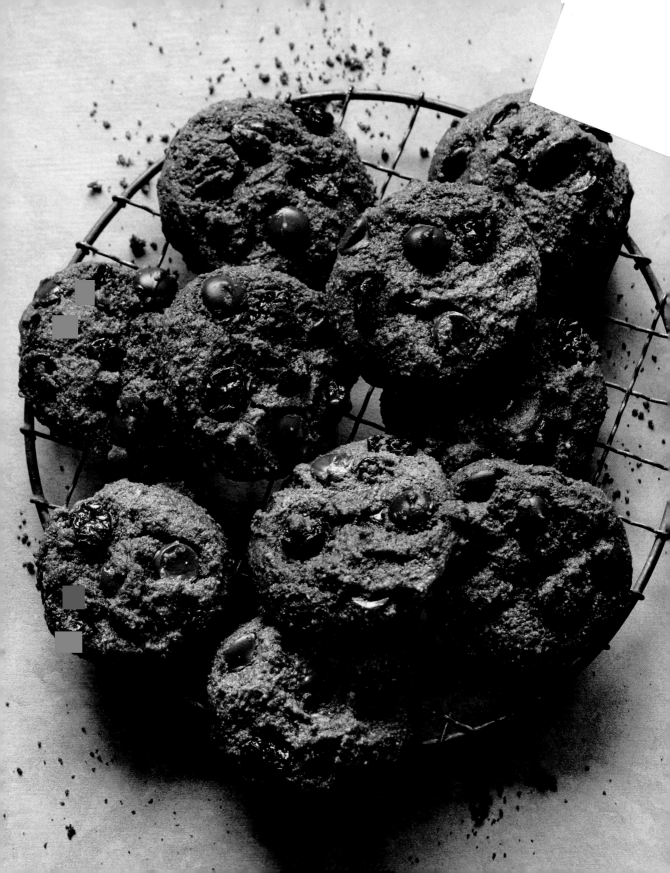

# FLOURLESS CHOCOLATE CHIP BLONDIES

YIELD: 12 BLONDIES | COOK TIME: 25 MINUTES

Olive oil spray

1 **15-oz can white beans,** drained and rinsed

7 **tbsp natural, no-salt-added peanut butter**

1 **tbsp virgin coconut oil,** melted

⅓ **cup granulated sugar**

1 **tsp vanilla extract**

2 **large egg whites**

1 **tbsp baking powder**

½ **tsp kosher salt**

½ **cup semisweet chocolate chips**

- Preheat the oven to 350°F.

- Spray a 9 x 9-inch pan with olive oil spray.

- Place the beans in the bowl of a food processor and puree until smooth; if necessary, add a tablespoon of water to help emulsify the beans.

- Turn off the food processor. Add the peanut butter, coconut oil, sugar, vanilla, egg whites, baking powder, and salt and blend until smooth. Scrape down the sides of the food processor to make sure that all of the ingredients are incorporated.

- Scrape the batter into the prepared pan.

- Sprinkle with the chocolate chips.

- Bake, uncovered, for 20 to 25 minutes, or until golden brown and the edges begin to loosen slightly from the pan.

- Transfer the pan to a baking rack to cool. Refrigerate for at least 1 hour or overnight. Slice into 12 portions and serve chilled.

**PER BLONDIE:** 165 calories / 9 g fat / 15 g carb / 4 g fiber / 6 g protein

# CHOCOLATE-COVERED STRAWBERRIES

YIELD: 20 STRAWBERRIES   COOK TIME: 5 MINUTES

**6** **oz semisweet chocolate**
(chips or bar)

**20** **strawberries,**
stems left on, rinsed,
and blotted dry

**20** **toothpicks**

- Place the chocolate chips in a microwave-safe bowl and microwave until melted. Stir every 30 seconds. Set aside to cool slightly.

- Line a plate or a rimmed baking sheet with parchment paper.

- Insert a toothpick into the stem of each strawberry. Dip the strawberries in the melted chocolate, turning to coat.

- Place the dipped strawberries on the lined plate and refrigerate until the chocolate hardens, about 20 minutes. Serve chilled.

**PER STRAWBERRY:** 138 calories / 3 g fat / 29 g carb / 7 g fiber / 2 g protein

# NO-CRUST PUMPKIN PIE

SERVES: 10 COOK TIME: 1 HOUR

Olive oil spray

2 eggs

1 15-oz can pure pumpkin puree

¾ cup (packed) light brown sugar

1 tsp ground cinnamon

½ tsp ground ginger

¼ tsp ground nutmeg

½ tsp kosher salt

1½ tsp vanilla extract

1 14-oz can full-fat, unsweetened coconut milk

1 cup Whipped Coconut Cream (page 188) (optional)

• Preheat the oven to 350°F. Spray a 9-inch oven-proof pie pan or 9 x 9-inch baking dish with olive oil spray.

• In a large bowl, whisk together the eggs, pumpkin, brown sugar, cinnamon, ginger, nutmeg, salt, and vanilla. Mix to combine. Add the coconut milk and whisk until smooth. Pour the mixture into the prepared pie pan.

• Bake in the oven for 1 hour, or until the center of the pie is firm and light golden brown.

• Transfer to a baking rack to cool for 1 hour and then place in the fridge. Refrigerate for at least 3 hours before slicing. Serve with a dollop of Whipped Coconut Cream if using.

**PER SERVING:** 170 calories / 6 g fat / 24 g carb / 2 g fiber / 3 g protein

# WATERMELON WEDGES with WHIPPED COCONUT CREAM, WALNUTS, and MINT

SERVES: 4    COOK TIME: N/A

¼  **large watermelon, sliced into wedges**

1  **lime**

¾  **cup Whipped Coconut Cream** (page 188)

¼  **cup raw walnuts,** toasted in a dry pan over medium heat until fragrant (about 2 minutes) and coarsely chopped

2  **tbsp coarsely chopped fresh mint leaves**

- Divide the watermelon wedges among four individual plates. Squeeze the lime on top of the watermelon. Place one-quarter of the Whipped Coconut Cream atop each wedge. Sprinkle each serving with 1 tablespoon toasted walnuts and garnish with mint.

**PER SERVING:** 135 calories / 5 g fat / 22 g carb / 2 g fiber / 2 g protein

# CHAPTER NINE

# ZERO BELLY DRINKS

Perfect Nutrition in a Glass—
Ready in Ninety Seconds or Less!

S imple, immediate, and stress-free: If you can create something that meets all three criteria and still delivers the goods, you've got a winner. And that's why I love ZERO BELLY Drinks.

These smoothies pack a perfect dose of nutrition—fiber, protein, and healthy fat, plus tons of vitamins, minerals, and other nutrients—into an incredibly simple meal (or snack, or even dessert) that goes from a gleam in your eye to a perfect meal in your glass in just minutes.

The recipes in these pages have been tested for their nutritional impact as well as their crave-worthy flavor. But you should consider them a blueprint for your own creative impulses. Just remember that before you build any smoothie, ask the three ZERO BELLY questions:

- **Where's my protein?**
- **Where's my fiber?**
- **Where's my healthy fat?**

With these recipes, the answer will always be—right here in your glass!

# FRESH BLUEBERRY (pictured)

SERVES: 1     COOK TIME: N/A

½   **cup unsweetened almond milk**

1   **scoop vanilla plant-based protein powder**

½   **cup frozen blueberries**

1½  **tsp natural, no-salt-added almond butter**

**Water to blend** (optional)

- Combine all of the ingredients in a blender and blend until smooth.

**PER SERVING:** 232 calories / 6 g fat / 16 g carb / 3 g fiber / 28 g protein

# STRAWBERRY BANANA

SERVES: 1     COOK TIME: N/A

½   **cup unsweetened almond milk**

1   **scoop vanilla plant-based protein powder**

⅓   **cup frozen strawberries**

¼   **frozen banana**

1½  **tsp natural, no-salt-added almond butter**

**Water to blend** (optional)

- Combine all of the ingredients in a blender and blend until smooth.

**PER SERVING:** 232 calories / 5 g fat / 18 g carb / 4 g fiber / 29 g protein

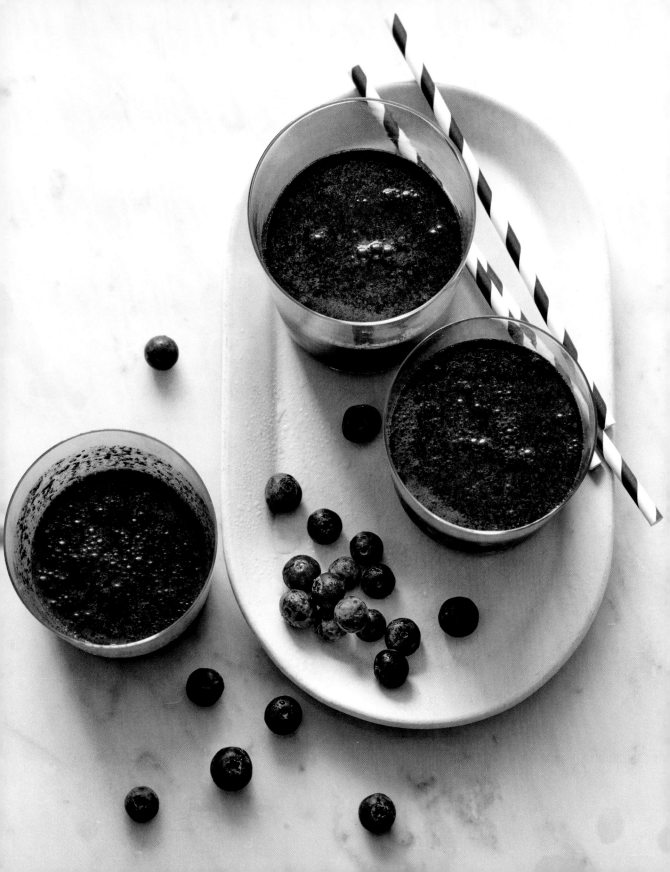

# PEANUT BUTTER CUP

SERVES: 1  COOK TIME: N/A

½ **cup unsweetened almond milk**

1 **scoop vanilla or chocolate plant-based protein powder**

1 **tbsp unsweetened cocoa powder** (non-alkalized)

½ **frozen banana**

1½ **tsp natural, no-salt-added peanut butter**

**Water to blend** (optional)

- Combine all of the ingredients in a blender and blend until smooth.

**PER SERVING:** 258 calories / 6 g fat / 21 g carb / 5 g fiber / 30 g protein

# MANGO ISLAND

SERVES: 1  COOK TIME: N/A

½ **cup unsweetened almond milk**

1 **scoop vanilla plant-based protein powder**

⅔ **cup frozen mango chunks**

1½ **tsp natural, no-salt-added almond butter**

**Water to blend** (optional)

- Combine all of the ingredients in a blender and blend until smooth.

**PER SERVING:** 224 calories / 5 g fat / 16 g carb / 3 g fiber / 29 g protein

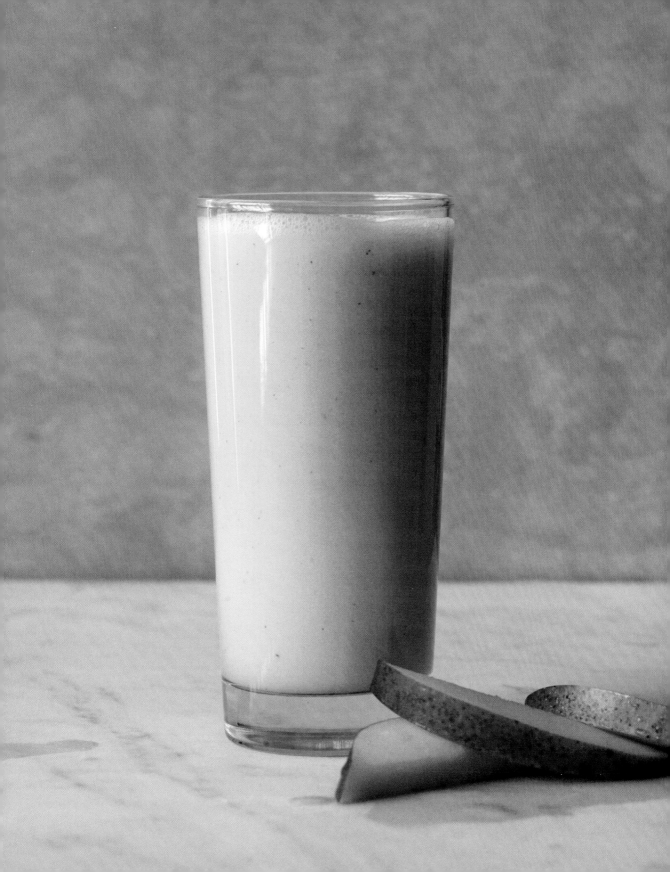

# VANILLA MILKSHAKE

SERVES: 1   COOK TIME: N/A

- ½  **cup unsweetened almond milk**
- 1  **scoop vanilla plant-based protein powder**
- ½  **frozen banana**
- 1½  **tsp natural, no-salt-added peanut butter**
- **Water to blend** (optional)

- Combine all of the ingredients in a blender and blend until smooth.

**PER SERVING:** 248 calories / 6 g fat / 20 g carb / 3 g fiber / 29 g protein

# GREEN MONSTER

SERVES: 1   COOK TIME: N/A

- ¼  **cup no-sugar-added apple juice**
- ¼  **cup water**
- ½  **scoop vanilla plant-based protein powder**
- ½  **Bosc pear,** chopped
- ½  **cup baby spinach,** loosely packed
- ½  **frozen banana**
- ¼  **ripe avocado**
- **Water to blend** (optional)

- Combine all of the ingredients in a blender and blend until smooth.

**PER SERVING:** 271 calories / 6 g fat / 40 g carb / 8 g fiber / 15 g protein

# VANILLA CHAI

SERVES: 1    COOK TIME: N/A

- ¼ **cup unsweetened almond milk**
- ¼ **cup chai tea** (brewed from a tea bag and chilled)
- ½ **scoop vanilla plant-based protein powder**
- ½ **frozen banana**
- ½ **tsp ground cinnamon**
- 1½ **tsp natural, no-salt-added almond butter**

  **Water to blend** (optional)

- • Combine all of the ingredients in a blender and blend until smooth.

**PER SERVING:** 219 calories / 9 g fat / 20 g carb / 4 g fiber / 17 g protein

# SUPERFOOD BOOSTER

SERVES: 1    COOK TIME: N/A

- ½ **cup unsweetened almond milk**

  **Juice of 1 large orange**
- ½ **scoop vanilla plant-based protein powder**
- ½ **frozen banana**
- 1½ **tsp raw Manuka honey** (optional)
- 1½ **tsp chia seeds,** soaked in water overnight
- ¼ **ripe avocado**

  **Water to blend** (optional)

- • Combine all of the ingredients in a blender and blend until smooth.

**PER SERVING:** 265 calories / 9 g fat / 31 g carb / 6 g fiber / 17 g protein

# PIÑA COLADA

½  cup light coconut milk

½  scoop vanilla plant-based protein powder

½  cup diced pineapple (fresh, frozen, or canned in juice)

¼  frozen banana

2  leaves fresh basil

   Water to blend (optional)

- Combine all of the ingredients in a blender and blend until smooth.

**PER SERVING:** 205 calories / 7 g fat / 21 g carb / 2 g fiber / 14 g protein

# CHOCOLATE DECADENCE

½  cup unsweetened almond milk

½  scoop plant-based chocolate protein powder

½  frozen banana

¼  ripe avocado

1  tbsp unsweetened cocoa powder (non-alkalized)

   Water to blend (optional)

- Combine all of the ingredients in a blender and blend until smooth.

**PER SERVING:**: 219 calories / 9 g fat / 20 g carb / 4 g fiber / 17 g protein

# GREEN MATCHA TEA

- ½ cup coconut water
- ½ scoop vanilla plant-based protein powder
- ½ cup baby spinach, loosely packed
- ½ frozen banana
- 1 tsp Matcha green tea powder
- 1 tsp ground cinnamon

  Water to blend (optional)

- Combine all of the ingredients in a blender and blend until smooth.

**PER SERVING:** 160 calories / 1 g fat / 25 g carb / 2 g fiber / 14 g protein

# BURMESE GIN THOKE
# MELON SALAD *by Susan Feniger*

SERVES: 12   COOK TIME: 40 MINUTES

½ **small seedless watermelon** (2½ pounds)

½ **ripe cantaloupe melon** (1½ pounds)

¼ **ripe honeydew melon** (1 pound)

2 **3-inch "thumbs" of young ginger,** finely minced (⅓ cup)

¼ **cup sesame seeds,** toasted

¼ **cup fresh lime juice** (3 to 4 limes)

¼ **cup low-sodium tamari**

½ **cup extra-virgin olive oil**

2 **tbsp plus 1 tsp granulated sugar**

1¾ **tsp kosher salt**

1 **cup green lentils**

1 **qt water**

1¼ **cups raw blanched peanuts**

2 **cups unsweetened flaked coconut**

4 **kaffir lime leaves,** chopped

- Start by cutting the melon. Trim off all of the rind for all three melons, remove any seeds, and cut into a ½-inch dice. Place all of the melon together in a large bowl and set aside.

- In a separate large bowl combine the ginger, sesame seeds, lime juice, tamari, ¼ cup olive oil, 2 tablespoons sugar, and ½ teaspoon salt. Mix well and pour over the melon.

- Toss and let marinate at room temperature while you prepare the rest of the salad.

- Put the lentils and water in a small saucepan over high heat. Bring to a boil (this takes about 5 minutes). Reduce the heat to low and simmer for 15 minutes more. Add 1 teaspoon salt and cook for 5 minutes more, or until the lentils are tender but not mushy.

- Drain and rinse the lentils with cold water to chill and then add to the melon mix. Stir and set aside.

- Mix the peanuts, coconut, kaffir lime leaves, the remaining 1 teaspoon of sugar, the remaining ¼ teaspoon of salt, and the remaining ¼ cup olive oil.

- Toast the peanut mixture in a large sauté pan over medium-low heat for 3 to 4 minutes, stirring constantly. The coconut and peanuts will toast, somewhat unevenly, to a golden brown.

- Remove from the heat and set aside to cool. Just before serving, add the peanut mixture to the melon mix and stir gently to combine.

- Serve in a large bowl, preferably at room temperature.

**PER SERVING:** 346 calories / 25 g fat / 25 g carb / 8 g fiber / 10 g protein

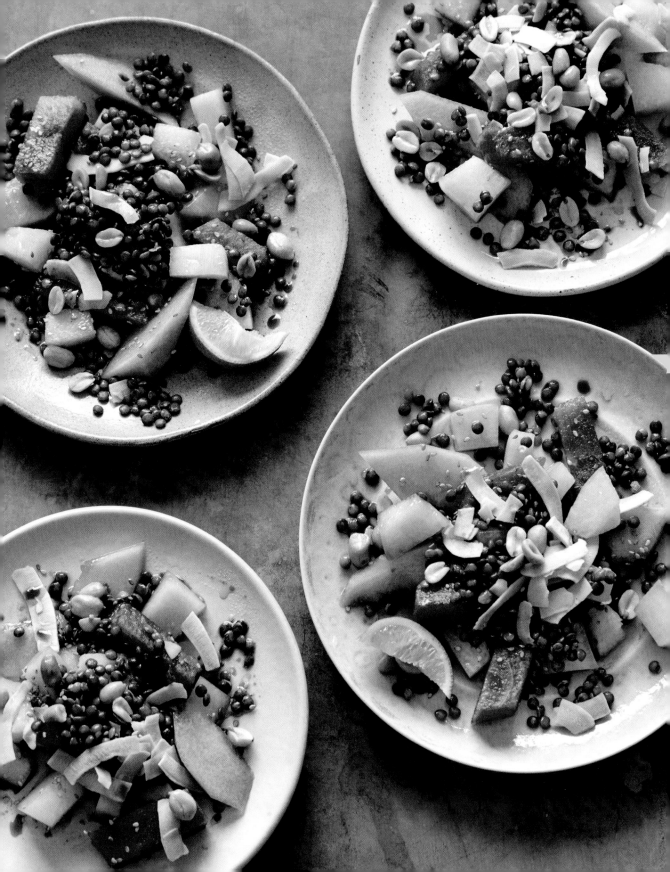

# PUMPKIN SOUP *by Chris Jaeckle*

SERVES: 4    COOK TIME: 10 MINUTES

1   tbsp extra-virgin olive oil

6   raw shrimp heads

2   cinnamon sticks, small

1   star anise

2   cloves

½   tsp mustard seeds

¼   tsp fennel seeds

¼   tsp cumin seeds

½   tsp coriander seeds

½   cup finely chopped shallot

4   tsp minced garlic

¼   cup minced fresh ginger

4½  lbs pumpkin, peeled and diced (about 1 small pumpkin)

1   qt water

1   qt low-sodium chicken broth

Sherry vinegar to taste

Kosher salt to taste

Granulated sugar to taste

- Heat the olive oil in a large pot over medium heat and roast shrimp heads, about 5 minutes.

- Remove heads from pan and set aside.

- Add cinnamon, star anise, and cloves. Add the mustard seeds and sauté until they begin to pop. Add fennel seeds and cumin seeds until they become aromatic. Then add the coriander seeds.

- Add the roasted shrimp heads back into the pot with the shallot, garlic, and ginger. Sweat these until they become softened.

- Add the pumpkin and sweat until soft-ened. Add the water and chicken broth.

- Cook until tender. Press through a china cap or mesh strainer.

- Season to taste with sherry vinegar, salt, and sugar.

**PER SERVING:** 196 calories / 4 g fat / 36 g carb / 3 g fiber / 6 g protein

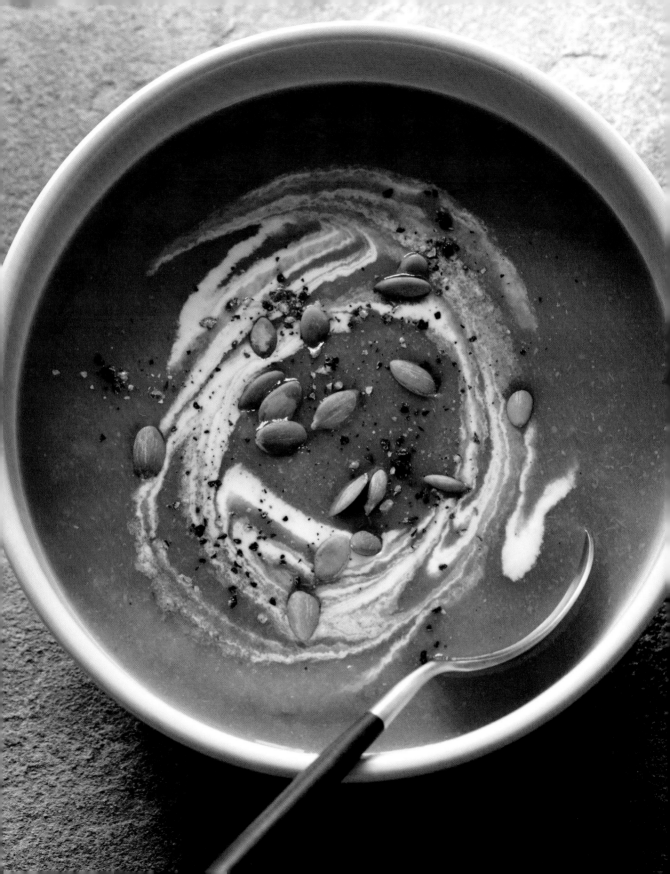

# AGUA CHILE *by Susan Feniger*

1 cucumber

½ bunch fresh cilantro

2 serrano peppers

¼ cup fresh lime juice

1 tsp salt

1 avocado

1 mango

2 Persian cucumbers

¾ lb Alaskan red king crab meat,
or lump crab meat

- Puree the cucumber, cilantro, serranos, lime juice, and salt together in a blender, then strain.

- Dice the avocado, mango, and Persian cucumbers into ½-inch dice.

- Divide the crab meat into 4 martini glasses or shallow bowls, then pour the agua chile over the top.
Finish with equal portions of avocado, mango, and Persian cucumber.

**PER SERVING:** 157 calories / 2 g fat / 21 g carb / 3 g fiber / 16 g protein

# CURRIED CHICKEN with RAISINS and CASHEW PUREE on GLUTEN-FREE BREAD *by Anita Lo*

SERVES: 4    COOK TIME: 25 MINUTES

1    **lb chicken tenders**

**Salt and freshly ground black pepper**

3    **tbsp extra-virgin olive oil**

½    **cup onion,** finely diced

1    **tbsp madras curry powder** (or to taste)

2    **tbsp raisins**

1    **pinch of grated lemon zest** (optional)

½    **tsp fresh lemon juice**

1    **tbsp chopped fresh chives** (optional)

*Cashew Puree*

⅓    **cup roasted salted cashews**

¼    **cup water**

**Salt and freshly ground black pepper to taste**

8    **slices gluten-free bread**

1    **Kirby cucumber,** cut into ¼-inch-thick rounds

**Lettuce**

- Season the chicken tenders with salt and pepper on both sides.

- Heat a small saucepan over high heat and add the olive oil. Add the onion and stir. Reduce the heat to medium and cook, stirring occasionally, until browned and very soft. Add the curry powder and stir. Add the seasoned chicken tenders and just cover with water. Raise the heat to medium-high and boil until the chicken tenders are cooked through, about 4 minutes.

- Transfer the cooked tenders to a bowl and continue to cook the remaining liquid until about 3 tablespoons remain. Pour over the tenders and allow to cool. Tear the cooked tenders into bite-size chunks and mix with the raisins, lemon zest, lemon juice, chives (if using), onion, and reduced liquid. Taste and adjust the seasonings.

- Make the cashew puree: With a hand blender or small blender, puree the cashews with the water and season to taste with salt and pepper.

- Lightly toast the bread, then spread with the cashew puree and line with cucumber slices and lettuce. Pile the curried chicken mixture in between and top with the other slice of bread.

**PER SERVING:** 497 calories / 23 g fat / 49 g carb / 9 g fiber / 26 g protein

# GRILLED FILLET of SWORDFISH with AVOCADO, GRAPEFRUIT, and CHILIES *by Anita Lo*

SERVES: 2    COOK TIME: 10 MINUTES

- **2 5-oz fillets of swordfish**
- **Salt and freshly ground black pepper**
- **2 tbsp extra-virgin olive oil**
- **1 pink grapefruit,** sectioned
- **1 avocado,** cut into bite-size pieces
- **2 tbsp fresh lime juice**
- **1 Thai bird chili,** finely chopped (substitute ½ serrano or jalapeño) or to taste
- **2 tbsp diced red onion**
- **2 tbsp roasted salted pistachios,** shelled
- **Salt and freshly ground black pepper to taste**

- Heat a grill or grill pan over high heat (you may broil instead if you don't have either). Season the fish with salt and pepper and rub with the olive oil. Grill to the desired temperature.

- Mix the remaining ingredients together. Taste and adjust the seasoning. Divide among two plates and serve the grilled fish on top.

**PER SERVING:** 562 calories / 42 g fat / 22 g carb / 9 g fiber / 37 g protein

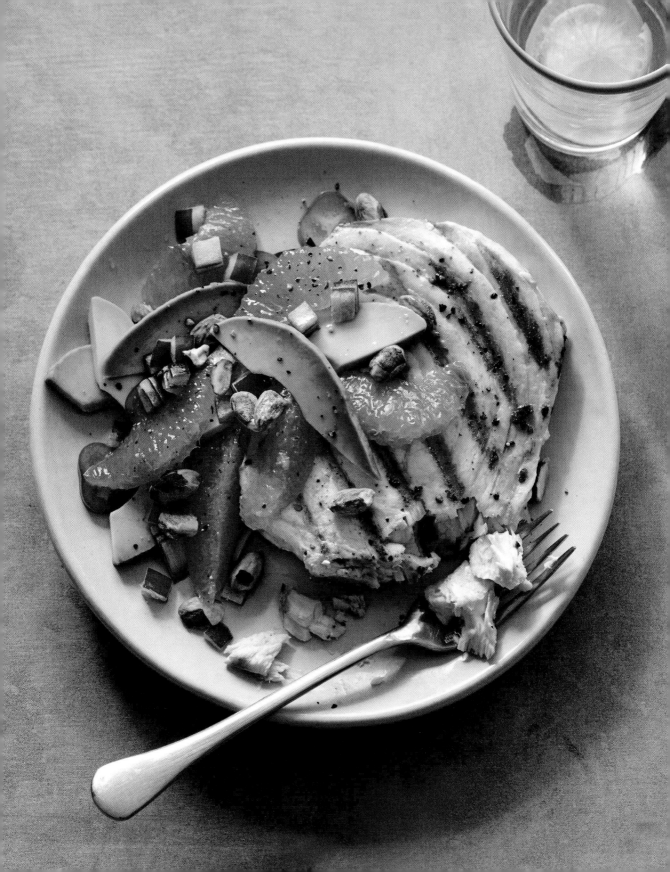

# WHOLE SNAPPER STUFFED with FENNEL and FENNEL SALAD *by Seamus Mullen*

**SERVES: 6    COOK TIME: 25 MINUTES**

1   **3-lb whole red snapper,** scaled, gutted, and gills removed

**Salt and freshly ground black pepper**

2   **bulbs fennel**

2   **blood oranges**

2   **tbsp unsalted butter**

1   **sprig fresh tarragon,** coarsely chopped

1   **sprig fresh mint,** coarsely chopped

2½   **tbsp extra-virgin olive oil**

1   **tsp white wine vinegar**

1   **lemon,** sliced

**Handful of fresh basil leaves**

**PER SERVING:**
357 calories /13 g fat /
12 g carb /3 g fiber /
48 g protein

- Season the snapper inside and out with salt and pepper and set aside.

- Cut one of the fennel bulbs in half and then each half again into four wedges. Juice one of the blood oranges and cut the other into supremes (sections).

- In a medium sauté pan, heat the butter over medium-high heat until it begins to foam, then add the fennel sections and gently brown for about 2 minutes on each side. Season with salt and pepper.

- Add the blood orange juice, reduce the heat, and braise the fennel until tender and cooked through, about 10 minutes. Set aside to cool.

- Preheat the oven to 425°F.

- For the fennel salad, thinly slice the remaining fennel with a mandoline or a very sharp knife and toss with the blood orange sections and the herbs and season with salt and pepper. Dress lightly with 1½ teaspoons olive oil and a drizzle of vinegar and set aside.

- Once the oven is preheated, stuff the braised fennel inside the cavity of the snapper. With a very sharp knife, score the skin of the fish three times on each side and carefully slip a slice of lemon into each score.

- Drizzle the fish with 1 tablespoon olive oil and roast in the oven until it is cooked through and reads 130°F with a meat thermometer or is hot at the thickest piece of the fillet when checked with a cake tester. This should take 12 to 15 minutes, depending on the size of the fish.

- Serve on a large platter on top of a bed of the shaved fennel salad with a squeeze of fresh lemon and the remaining tablespoon of olive oil. Enjoy immediately.

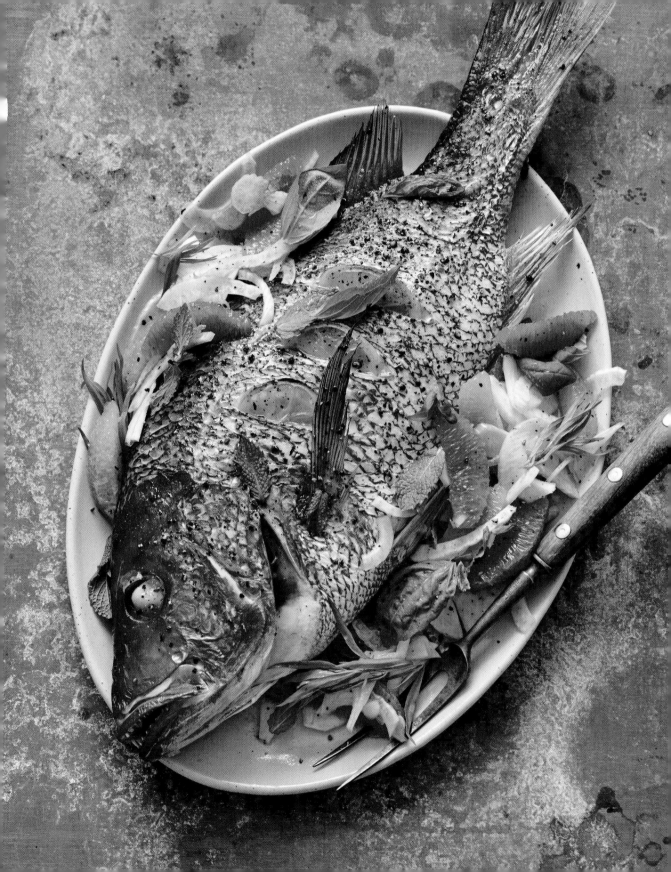

# TSUMI TUNA TEMAKI
## by Chris Jaeckle

**SERVES: 1    COOK TIME: 25 MINUTES**

- ½ **cup cooked sushi rice** (recipe follows)
- 1 **nori sheet**
- 1 **tbsp fresh tuna,** sliced
- ¼ **tbsp kizami wasabi mix** (recipe follows)
- ½ **tbsp green apple slices**

- Spread rice on the left half of the nori. Top the rice with the tuna, kizami wasabi, and apple slices and roll into a cone shape.

### Sushi Rice
- 2 **cups rice**
- 2 **cups water**
- ⅓ **cup rice wine vinegar**

### Special Equipment
- **Rice cooker**

- Wash rice until the water runs clear. Then drain. Add the water and rice to a rice cooker. Cook until the rice cooker switches to hold mode. Leave covered for 15 minutes. Remove the rice and place it in a large bowl. Fan the rice until just above body temperature and drizzle the vinegar over the rice. Toss gently.

### Kizami Wasabi
- ⅓ **cup extra-virgin olive oil**
- 1 **cup scallion whites,** minced
- 2 **tbsp fresh ginger,** minced
- 1 **cup kizami wasabi**
- 1 **tbsp rice wine vinegar**

- Heat the olive oil in a pan. Add the scallions and ginger. Sweat for 3 to 5 minutes, until the scallions are softened but not translucent. Add the kizami wasabi and rice vinegar. Stir to incorporate and cool immediately.

**PER SERVING:** 305 calories / 2 g fat / 53 g carb / 3 g fiber / 12 g protein

*My Zero Belly temaki combines the earthy bite of kizami wasabi, the spicy tang of ginger, and the mouthwatering tartness of green apple slices— all rolled up around one of the most powerful Zero Belly foods: lean tuna. Yum.*

— **CHRIS JAECKLE,** EXECUTIVE CHEF, ALL'ONDA

# PREP-AHEAD RECIPES
## Dressings, Sauces, Marinades, and Dips

## ZERO BELLY VINAIGRETTE

YIELD: ½ CUP  COOK TIME: N/A

- 3 tbsp raw apple cider vinegar
- ⅓ cup extra-virgin olive oil
- ¾ tsp Dijon mustard
- ¾ tsp raw Manuka honey*
- ⅛ tsp kosher salt
- ⅛ tsp freshly ground black pepper

- Combine the ingredients in a glass jar and shake vigorously until emulsified. Store in the fridge for up to 2 weeks. Shake before serving.

**PER TBSP:** 83 calories / 9 g fat / 1 g carb / 0 g fiber / 0 g protein

## ASIAN SALAD DRESSING

YIELD: ½ CUP  COOK TIME: N/A

- ⅓ cup rice wine vinegar
- 3 tbsp extra-virgin olive oil
- 2 tbsp raw Manuka honey*
- 2 tbsp low-sodium tamari

- Combine the ingredients in a glass jar and shake vigorously until emulsified. Store in the fridge for up to 2 weeks. Shake before serving.

If the honey is solid, heat the jar (metal lid removed) in the microwave for 30 seconds. The dressing may congeal slightly in the fridge.

**PER TBSP:** 88 calories / 5 g fat / 10 g carb / 0 g fiber / 0 g protein

# RED-HOT BUFFALO DRESSING

YIELD: ½ CUP   COOK TIME: N/A

- 3 tbsp hot sauce
- ¼ cup Zero Belly Mayonnaise (page 242)
- 2 tbsp Zero Belly Vinaigrette (page 236)

- Combine the ingredients in a glass jar and shake vigorously until emulsified. Store in the fridge for up to 2 weeks. Shake before serving.

The dressing may congeal slightly in the fridge.

**PER TBSP:** 52 calories / 6 g fat / 0 g carb / 0 g fiber / 0 g protein

# ITALIAN DRESSING

YIELD: ½ CUP   COOK TIME: N/A

- ⅓ cup extra-virgin olive oil
- 2 tbsp white wine vinegar
- 1 tbsp Dijon mustard
- 1 tbsp fresh lemon juice
- 2 cloves garlic, minced
- 1 tbsp dried basil
- 1 tbsp dried oregano

- Combine the ingredients in a glass jar and shake vigorously until emulsified. Store in the fridge for up to 2 weeks. Shake before serving.

**PER TBSP:** 83 calories / 9 g fat / 0 g carb / 0 g fiber / 0 g protein

# ZERO BELLY SOFRITO

YIELD: 1 CUP    COOK TIME: 8 MINUTES

Sofrito is a base sauce used in Spanish, Portuguese, and Latin American cooking. Preparations may vary, but it typically consists of aromatic ingredients cut into small pieces and sautéed in oil. This version uses ginger, a hot chili pepper, and extra-virgin olive oil—ingredients proven to target belly fat. You'll use this simple sauce as a base for many recipes in the cookbook. Consider it extra-virgin olive oil with a Zero Belly kick!

| | |
|---|---|
| 1 | serrano chili |
| ⅓ | cup coarsely chopped shallots (about 2 large or 3 small) |
| ⅓ | cup coarsely chopped fresh ginger |
| ½ | cup extra-virgin olive oil |

- Take the stem off of the chili and cut the chili in half. Take the seeds out and slice thin. Place the chili, shallots, and ginger in the bowl of a food processor and chop until finely minced.

- Heat the oil in a saucepan over medium heat and add the shallots, ginger, and chilies.

- Reduce the heat to low and cook until the shallots and aromatics are very soft, about 8 minutes.

- Remove from the heat and cool.

- Store in a glass jar in the fridge for up to 1 week.

Sofrito may congeal slightly in the fridge. For recipes that call for removing oil first, heat the jar (metal lid removed) in the microwave for 30 seconds.

**PER TBSP:** 63 calories / 7 g fat / 1 g carb / 0 g fiber / 0 g protein

# BLACK PEPPER MARINADE

**YIELD: 1 CUP COOK TIME: N/A**

- **2** tbsp whole coriander seeds
- **2** tbsp whole black peppercorns
- **½** tbsp whole cumin seeds
- **6** cloves garlic, peeled
- **1** 1-inch piece of fresh ginger, peeled and sliced thin
- **3** shallots, peeled and sliced thin
- **¼** cup extra-virgin olive oil
- **¼** cup (packed) brown sugar

- Grind the coriander seeds, peppercorns, and cumin seeds in a spice grinder or clean coffee grinder until very fine.

- Add the remaining ingredients to the bowl of a small food processor and puree until smooth. Add the ground spices and process to incorporate.

- Store in a glass jar in the fridge for up to 1 week.

**PER TBSP:** 47 calories / 3 g fat / 4 g carb / 0 g fiber / 0 g protein

# MEXICAN SPICE BLEND

YIELD: ½ CUP   COOK TIME: N/A

2½ tbsp chili powder

1 tsp kosher salt

4 tsp paprika

2 tsp ground cumin

4 tsp onion powder

4 tsp garlic powder

- Mix the spices in a small bowl to combine.

- Store in a glass jar away from direct sunlight for up to 1 month.

**PER TBSP:** 83 calories / 9 g fat / 1 g carb / 0 g fiber / 0 g protein

# ARUGULA CHIMICHURRI

YIELD: 1 CUP   COOK TIME: N/A

¾ cup packed baby arugula (about 1 oz)

½ bunch fresh parsley

¼ cup Zero Belly Sofrito (page 238)

3 tbsp red wine vinegar

2 cloves garlic, minced

¼ tsp kosher salt

¼ tsp freshly ground black pepper

- Place the arugula and parsley in the bowl of a food processor. Pulse until well chopped. Add the rest of the ingredients and pulse until well incorporated but still chunky.

- Serve immediately, or store in a glass jar in the fridge for up to 1 week

**PER TBSP:** 26 calories / 2.5 g fat / 1 g carb / 0 g fiber / 0 g protein

# MARINARA

- **1 small onion
  or ½ large onion,**
  finely chopped

- **4 cloves garlic,**
  minced

- **1 tbsp extra-virgin
  olive oil**

- **2 cups canned crushed
  tomatoes with the juice**

- **½ tsp dried rosemary**

- **½ tsp dried thyme leaves**

- **¼ cup Kalamata olives,**
  halved, pits removed

- **½ tsp kosher salt**

- **¼ cup water**
  (optional)

- **1 bunch fresh basil,**
  picked of stems and
  coarsely chopped

- In a medium saucepan, add the onion, garlic, and olive oil and cook, stirring occasionally, over medium heat, until the onion starts to soften, about 3 minutes.

- Add the tomatoes, rosemary, thyme, olives, and salt and simmer for 5 minutes. Add the water to thin the sauce to your preference.

- Remove from the heat and stir in the basil.

- Serve immediately or store in a glass container in the fridge for up to 1 week.

**PER ½ CUP:** 100 calories / 5 g fat / 12 g carb / 1 g fiber / 2 g protein

## TO

- 2½  **cups packed fresh basil leaves,** rinsed and dried
- 3  **cloves garlic,** coarsely chopped
- ⅓  **cup raw pecans,** toasted in a dry pan over medium heat until fragrant (about 2 minutes)
- 1  **tsp kosher salt**
- ½  **cup extra-virgin olive oil**

- Place all of the pesto ingredients except the olive oil in the bowl of a food processor. Pulse for a few seconds. Then turn on the processor and pour in the olive oil in a steady stream, until the pesto reaches the right consistency: pureed and not too chunky.

- Serve immediately or store in a BPA-free container in the fridge for up to 1 week.

**PER TBSP:** 78 calories / 8 g fat / 1 g carb / 0 g fiber / 0 g protein

# ZERO BELLY MAYONNAISE

- 2  **egg yolks**
  **Juice of 1 lemon**
- ½  **tsp Dijon mustard**
- ¼  **tsp kosher salt**
- 1  **cup extra-virgin olive oil**

- Place all of the mayonnaise ingredients except the olive oil in the bowl of a food processor. Pulse for a few seconds. Then turn on the processor and pour in the olive oil in a steady stream, allowing the mayonnaise to emulsify.

- Serve immediately or store in a BPA-free container in the fridge for up to 10 days.

If you've never tried homemade mayonnaise, you're missing out! This version uses only the freshest, purest ingredients. Make it your own by adding your favorite fresh herbs and Zero Belly spices.

**PER TBSP:** 84 calories / 9 g fat / 0 g carb / 0 g fiber / 0 g protein

# TARTAR SAUCE

YIELD: ½ CUP | COOK TIME: N/A

- ½ cup **Zero Belly Mayonnaise** (page 242)
- 3 **tbsp relish**
- 2 **tbsp fresh lemon juice**

- Whisk together the ingredients in a small bowl.
- Serve immediately or store in a BPA-free container in the fridge for up to 10 days.

**PER TBSP:** 64 calories / 7 g fat / 1 g carb / 0 g fiber / 0 g protein

# GUACAMOLE

YIELD: 3 CUPS | COOK TIME: N/A

- 3 **avocados,** halved, pit removed, peeled, and cubed
- 1 **tsp kosher salt**
  **Juice of 1 lime**
- ½ **cup red onion,** finely diced
- 2 **tsp ground cumin** (optional)
- 2 **plum tomatoes,** diced
- ¼ **cup coarsely chopped fresh cilantro**

- Add the avocado, salt, and fresh lime juice in a medium bowl. Use the back of a fork to smash the ingredients together until lumpy. Stir in the remaining ingredients with a rubber spatula. Serve immediately.

**PER ¼ CUP:** 64 calories / 6 g fat / 4 g carbs / 3 g fiber / 1 g protein

# HUMMUS

YIELD: 1½ CUPS   COOK TIME: N/A

1   **15-oz can garbanzo beans,** beans rinsed, canning liquid reserved

1   **tbsp lemon juice**

2   **tbsp extra-virgin olive oil**

1   **clove garlic,** coarsely chopped

½   **tsp kosher salt**

- Place the beans, lemon juice, olive oil, garlic, and salt in the bowl of a food processor. Pulse for a few seconds, turn on the processor, and then add some of the bean liquid, 1 tablespoon at a time, until smooth and creamy.

- Serve immediately, or store in a glass jar in the fridge for up to 1 week.

**PER ¼ CUP:** 120 calories / 6 g fat / 15 g carb / 4 g fiber / 4 g protein

# GREEN GODDESS DRESSING

YIELD: 1 CUP   COOK TIME: N/A

2   **cloves garlic**

1   **large avocado,** skin and pit removed

3   **tbsp raw apple cider vinegar**

**Juice of 1 lemon**

¼   **cup extra-virgin olive oil**

½   **cup fresh basil leaves,** packed

½   **cup fresh parsley,** packed

2   **scallions,** greens only

1   **tsp kosher salt**

- Place the garlic, avocado, vinegar, and lemon juice in the bowl a food processor and puree until smooth. While the food processor is running, add the olive oil in a steady stream, allowing the dressing to emulsify. Turn off the processor, add the herbs, scallions, and salt, and pulse until the herbs are finely chopped but maintain some texture. The dip will be slightly chunky.

- Serve immediately or store in a glass jar in the fridge for up to 4 days.

**PER ¼ CUP:** 101 calories / 10 g fat / 2 g carb / 2 g fiber / 1 g protein

# SALSA

YIELD: 2 CUPS   COOK TIME: N/A

5   **ripe plum tomatoes,** quartered

¼   **red onion,** thinly sliced

1   **jalapeño,** halved, veins and seeds removed

8   **sprigs fresh cilantro**

3   **cloves garlic,** crushed

**Juice of 1 lime**

- Place all of the ingredients in the bowl of a food processor and pulse until coarsely chopped.

- Serve immediately or store in a BPA-free container in the fridge for up to 4 days.

**PER 2 TBSP:** 5 calories / 0 g fat / 1 g carb / 0 g fiber / 0 g protein

# ROASTED RED PEPPER DIP

YIELD: 1 CUP   COOK TIME: N/A

½   **cup jarred roasted red peppers in water** (3 tbsp of water from jar reserved)

2   **cloves garlic,** peeled

3   **tbsp raw walnuts,** toasted in a dry pan over medium heat until fragrant (about 2 minutes)

2   **scallions, coarsely chopped**

¼   **cup extra-virgin olive oil**

1   **tbsp red wine vinegar**

¼   **tsp kosher salt**

¼   **tsp freshly ground black pepper**

- Place the roasted peppers and reserved water, garlic, walnuts, and scallions in the bowl of a food processor and puree until smooth. Add the olive oil, vinegar, salt, and pepper and puree until smooth.

- Serve immediately or store in a BPA-free container in the fridge for up to 4 days.

**PER ¼ CUP:** 84 calories / 9 g fat / 1 g carb / 1 g fiber / 1 g protein

# GRILLED CHICKEN BREAST

**SERVES: 4 | COOK TIME: 12 MINUTES**

**1 lb skinless, boneless chicken breasts**

**Olive oil spray**

**Kosher salt and freshly ground black pepper**

- Heat a grill or grill pan over medium heat.

- Spray the chicken lightly with olive oil spray, season both sides with a pinch of salt and pepper, and place on the grill.

- Allow the chicken to sit undisturbed until grill marks form, 3 to 4 minutes. Quarter-turn the breasts on the same side and cook for 3 to 4 minutes more. Turn the breasts over and repeat the two-step grilling process. Transfer the cooked chicken to a clean plate to cool.

- Serve immediately or store in a glass container in the fridge for up to 5 days.

**PER SERVING:** 171 calories / 4 g fat / 0 g carb / 0 g fiber / 35 g protein

# TURKEY MEATBALLS

1   **lb extra-lean ground turkey** (99%)

⅔   **cup Brown Rice** (page 253)

½   **tsp freshly ground black pepper**

2   **large egg whites**

¼   **cup Zero Belly Sofrito,** oil drained (page 238)

- Preheat the oven to 350°F.

- In a mixing bowl, combine the turkey, brown rice, pepper, egg whites, and sofrito and mix until well combined.

- Roll the mixture into 24 meatballs the size of a large marble (about 1 tablespoon each) and set on a rimmed baking sheet.

- Bake for 10 to 13 minutes, or until cooked through.

- Serve immediately or store in a glass container in the fridge for up to 5 days.

**PER SERVING:** 248 calories / 11 g fat / 9 g carb / 1 g fiber / 29 g protein

# OVEN-ROASTED WHITEFISH

SERVES: 4 | COOK TIME: 10 MINUTES

1 **lb whitefish**
such as halibut or
Pacific cod

**Olive oil spray**

**Salt and freshly ground
black pepper**

- Preheat the oven to 350°F.

- Place the fish on a nonstick rimmed baking sheet. Spray the fish lightly with olive oil spray and season on both sides with a pinch of salt and pepper. Place the baking sheet in the oven and cook for 6 to 8 minutes.

- Serve immediately or store the cooled fish in a glass container in the fridge for up to 3 days.

**PER SERVING:** 125 calories / 2 g fat / 0 g carb / 0 g fiber / 26 g protein

# SEARED TUNA

SERVES: 4 | COOK TIME: 10 MINUTES

1½ **tsp kosher salt**

1½ **tsp ground coriander**

1½ **tsp ground fennel seed**

1½ **tsp freshly ground
black pepper**

1 **tbsp extra-virgin olive oil**

1 **lb fresh Ahi tuna**

If you prefer a medium doneness, sear for 2 to 3 minutes on each side. If you prefer your tuna well-done, sear for 2 minutes on each side and finish cooking in a 350°F oven for 6 minutes.

- Combine the salt and spices in a small bowl. Sprinkle the tuna evenly with the spice mix and set aside to let marinate for 5 minutes.

- Place a nonstick pan over medium-high heat and add the olive oil. Once the olive oil is hot, add the tuna to the pan with a pair of tongs and let it sear, undisturbed, for 1 minute.*

- Flip the tuna over and sear for another minute. Transfer the tuna to a clean plate to cool. Serve immediately.

**PER SERVING:** 150 calories / 5 g fat / 0 g carb / 0 g fiber / 27 g protein

# GRILLED STEAK

**1  lb sirloin**

- Heat a grill or grill pan over medium-high heat.

- Place the steak(s) on the grill using a pair of tongs and let sit until marked, 3 to 4 minutes. Quarter-turn the steak on the same side and repeat, letting the steak sit undisturbed for 2 to 4 minutes.

- Turn the steaks over and let sit on the grill, undisturbed, for 3 to 4 minutes. Quarter-turn the steaks on the same side and let cook for 3 to 4 minutes more. Pull the steaks off the grill and let rest.

- Allow to rest for 5 minute before serving. Once cooled, store in a glass container in the fridge for up to 4 days.

**PER SERVING:** 150 calories / 5 g fat / 0 g carb / 0 g fiber / 27 g protein

# POACHED SHRIMP

**1  lb shrimp, fresh or defrosted,** heads removed, peeled, and deveined

- Bring a large saucepan of water to a boil.

- Meanwhile, prepare a large bowl of ice water.

- Add the shrimp to the saucepan, cover, and boil for 2 minutes. Using a slotted spoon, transfer the cooked shrimp to the ice water bath to cool. Transfer the shrimp to a plate covered with paper towels to dry.

- Serve immediately or store in a glass container in the fridge for up to 3 days.

**PER SERVING:** 107 calories / 1 g fat / 0 g carb / 0 g fiber / 24 g protein

# HARD-BOILED EGGS

**SERVES: 4  COOK TIME: 10 MINUTES**

**12  eggs**

- Place the eggs in a medium pot of cold water. Turn the heat on high and bring to a boil.

- Once the water boils, turn off the heat and let the eggs sit for 10 minutes in the hot water.

- Meanwhile, fill a large bowl with ice and cold water.

- Place the boiled eggs in the ice water using a slotted spoon. Let cool for 2 to 3 minutes. Once cool, crack each egg on a tabletop and use your fingers to peel the shell off. Rinse each egg in cold water to remove any remaining shell.

- Serve immediately or store in a glass container in the fridge for up to 1 week.

For soft-boiled eggs, boil eggs for 5 minutes before transferring to an ice water bath to cool.

**PER SERVING:** 150 calories / 5 g fat / 0 g carb / 0 g fiber / 27 g protein

# PREP-AHEAD RECIPES
## Grains, Legumes, and Vegetables

# QUINOA

YIELD: 3 CUPS   COOK TIME: 30 MINUTES

- 1 cup quinoa
- 2 cups cold water
- ½ tsp kosher salt

- Rinse the quinoa under cold water for 30 seconds. Drain and transfer to a medium saucepan.

- Add the water and salt and bring to a boil.

- Cover, reduce the heat to medium-low, and simmer until the water is absorbed, 15 to 20 minutes.

- Remove from the heat and let sit for 5 minutes. Uncover and fluff with a fork.

- Serve immediately or store in a glass container in the fridge for up to 1 week.

**PER ½ CUP:** 106 calories / 2 g fat / 20 g carb / 2 g fiber / 4 g protein

# QUINOA "STUFFING" with DRIED CHERRIES and WALNUTS

1  **large onion,**
   finely diced

2  **celery stalks,**
   finely diced

2  **tbsp extra-virgin
   olive oil**

1  **cup Quinoa,**
   cooked (page 251)

⅓  **cup raw walnuts,**
   toasted in a dry pan
   over medium heat
   until fragrant
   (about 2 minutes)

⅓  **cup dried tart cherries**

4  **sage leaves,**
   coarsely chopped
   (optional)

   **Kosher salt to taste**

- Sauté the onion, celery, and olive oil in a small pan over medium heat until tender, about 5 minutes.

- Place the sautéed vegetables, quinoa, walnuts, cherries, and sage in a large bowl and toss to combine. Add salt to taste.

- Divide among four plates.

- Serve alone, with Grilled Chicken Breast (page 246), or as a pre-cooked stuffing for Perfect Roast Chicken or Turkey (page 156).

**PER SERVING:** 349 calories / 16 g fat / 45 g carb / 5 g fiber / 8 g protein

# BROWN RICE

1  **cup long-grain brown rice**

2  **cups water**

½  **teaspoon salt**

- Place the rice in a fine-mesh strainer and rinse under cold water until the water runs clear.

- Place the measured water in a medium saucepan with a lid and bring to a boil over high heat.

- Add the rice and salt, stir to incorporate, cover, and reduce the heat to low.

- Simmer undisturbed until the rice is tender, 45 to 50 minutes.

- Remove from the heat and let sit covered to steam for 10 minutes more.

- Fluff with a fork and serve.

- Serve immediately or store in a glass container in the fridge for up to 1 week.

**PER ½ CUP:** 100 calories / 1 g fat / 22 g carb / 2 g fiber / 2 g protein

# GREEN LENTILS

YIELD: 2 CUPS    COOK TIME: 35 MINUTES

1   cup dried green lentils

2   cups water

1   bay leaf, clove garlic,
    or other seasoning

½   tsp salt

- Rinse the lentils in a colander and transfer to a saucepan. Cover with the water and the bay leaf, garlic, and any other seasonings. Reserve the salt.

- Bring the water to a rapid simmer over medium-high heat, then reduce the heat to maintain a very gentle simmer. Cook, uncovered, for 20 to 30 minutes. Add water as needed to make sure the lentils are just barely covered. The lentils are cooked as soon as they are tender and no longer crunch.

- Strain the lentils and remove the bay leaf or garlic.

- Return the lentils to the pan and stir in the salt.

- Serve immediately or store in a glass container in the fridge for up to 1 week.

TIP   Any amount of lentils can be cooked in this manner. Just maintain a 2:1 ratio of water to lentils.

**PER ½ CUP:** 115 calories / 1 g fat / 20 g carb / 8 g fiber / 9 g protein

# GRILLED MIXED VEGETABLES

YIELD: 4 CUPS   COOK TIME: 20 MINUTES

1 **large summer squash,** sliced into ¼-inch rounds

1 **large zucchini squash,** sliced into ¼-inch rounds

1 **small eggplant,** sliced into ⅓-inch rounds

1 **large head of fennel,** sliced into ¼-inch rounds

1 **bunch green asparagus** (about 12 spears), white part of stems removed

   **Olive oil spray**

- Heat a grill or grill pan over medium heat.

- Spray the prepared vegetables with olive oil spray.

- Using a pair of tongs, place the sliced squash on the grill and cook for 3 to 4 minutes per side, or until the slices are crisp and tender, with nicely browned grill marks. Transfer the squash to a plate or rimmed baking sheet to cool, and repeat with the remaining vegetables.

- Transfer all the cooked vegetables to a bowl and toss to combine.

- Serve immediately or store in a glass container in the fridge for up to 3 days.

**PER ½ CUP:** 65 calories / 1 g fat / 15 g carb / 7 g fiber / 4 g protein

# Acknowledgments

This book would not have been possible—not to mention nearly so delicious—without the creativity, hard work, patience, and highly attuned palates of the following team:

My co-author, Jason Lawless, who amazes me time and again with his inventive takes on food. He makes even everyday foods taste new, original, and extraordinary—every time.

Cecelia Smith, who coordinated this project and kept Jason and me on track to deliver what we truly believe is a revolutionary new plan with revolutionary new recipes.

Jason Varney, whose glorious photos somehow capture not just the sights but the scents, sounds, and flavors of these tantalizing recipes.

Gina Centrello, Libby McGuire, Marnie Cochran, Bill Takes, Richard Callison, Nina Shield, Joe Perez, Quinne Rogers, Susan Corcoran, Cindy Murray, and the entire team at Ballantine, whose passion for this project kept us hungry, even as we were cooking and writing into the wee hours.

Michael Freidson, George Karabotsos, Steve Perrine, Charlene Lutz, Jon Hammond, Sean Bumgarner, Ray Jobst, Lihn Le, Daniel McCarter, John Phelan, Linnea Zielinski, Dana Smith, Daniel Cohen, Jorge Olivares, and everyone else at Galvanized. You're empire builders, and I'm glad to be on board while you're changing the world.

Jennifer Rudolph Walsh, Jon Rosen, and the great folks at William Morris Endeavor.

Ben Sherwood, Barbara Fedida, and the team at ABC News.

Dan Abrams, Christine Cole, and the culinary superstars at White Street.

Larry Shire, Eric Sacks, and Jonathan Erlich, for their invaluable counsel.

Mehmet Oz, David Pecker, Dave Freygang, Steve Lacey, Strauss Zelnick, Steve Gilbert, Steve Murphy, Michele Promaulayko, and the many friends, colleagues, and advisers who continue to inspire us with their wisdom and insight.

Thanks, too, to the many fans of Zero Belly who not only tested these recipes, but created many of their own especially for this book.

And most important of all, this book is brought to you through the good graces and support of the best family a man could ever have.

# INDEX

Page references in *italics* refer to illustrations.